the Mommy Mojo Makeover

the Mommy Mojo Makeover

28 TOOLS TO RECLAIM YOURSELF & REIGNITE YOUR RELATIONSHIP

DANA B. MYERS

FOUNDER OF BOOTY PARLOR

V!VA
EDITIONS

Published in the United States by Viva Editions, an imprint of Start Midnight, LLC, 101 Hudson Street, Thirty-Seventh Floor, Suite 3705, Jersey City, NJ 07302.

Printed in the United States.
Cover design: Scott Idleman/Blink
Text design: Frank Wiedemann
First Edition.
10 9 8 7 6 5 4 3 2 1

Trade paper ISBN: 978-1-62778-282-1
E-book ISBN: 978-1-62778-283-8

Library of Congress Cataloging-in-Publication Data is available on file.

I dedicate this book to . . .
myself,
with love, pride, and sweet satisfaction.

This commitment was my compass;
a guide to becoming the mother, lover,
and woman I am today,
so that I could share this knowledge
with you, Mama.

TABLE OF CONTENTS

· · · · · · · · · · · · · ·

Motherhood, Marriage . . . and Mojo

HELLO, GORGEOUS . . . AND WELCOME TO THE MOMMY MOJO MAKEOVER!

I'M THRILLED YOU'VE DECIDED to take part in this transformational journey to reawakening your sexuality and reigniting the spark in your relationship. You are on your way to a sexier, more confident and satisfying experience of motherhood and partnership.

But, before we begin, I want to share a story with you: Several years ago, I was in Los Angeles, giving a blowjob workshop for an A-list celebrity and her friends. Yes, you read that right. As a sex expert and the founder of the sexy lifestyle brand Booty Parlor, I often do these types of things!

This celebrity had two children and was married to one of the most gorgeous leading men in Hollywood. When I walked in her front door, bag of cucumbers in hand, I took stock of her life: an amazing career, a stylish home, gorgeous children, and an insanely hot husband. When she met me at the door, she looked flushed and vibrant, like she'd just had an orgasm.

And I thought, *Yes! I want that! I can have that!*

At the time, I was six months pregnant with my first child. I spent my days running my business, zen-ning out in prenatal yoga classes, seeing girlfriends, going on fun dates and weekend trips with my husband, and shopping for the nursery. I daydreamed about the baby that was coming, imagining how I would effortlessly slide into my perfect vision of blissful, working motherhood and Pinterest-worthy domesticity. In those visions, I had it all: the career, the baby, the body that bounced back, the sizzling sex life. When I saw this celebrity mom looking stunning in her fabulous house with her darling children and hunky husband, it gave me the mental confirmation that I, too, could have it all.

But the glittering little vision I'd created was about to crack. As I demonstrated my best manhandling maneuvers in the workshop, amidst giggles, chitchat, and champagne sipping, the celebrity nodded and laughed and even took a few notes. But then, out of nowhere, her smile faded and she said, "I've got to be honest with you. I'm just not that into sex anymore. I'm so tired. And my libido? Well . . . it's dead. My husband's gorgeous and a great parent and I love him, but the lust is gone."

She pointed at my bulging belly, took a huge crunch out of her cucumber in the now-silent room, and said, "You'll see."

I was stunned silent. I thought, *Wait, what? I won't see. No, I can't see. That's just not an option for me!*

How could this be? My career—no, my *life*—was dedicated to empowering women to live a sexier, more turned-on lifestyle. Pursuing sensual pleasure and romance was my passion! It was second nature to me. Sex was always how I expressed myself; an outlet for my creativity, a playground to unleash my inner wild-girl, a channel to release my anxiety, frustration, and sadness. I couldn't imagine living without that energy, that desire, that electricity, that *Mojo* within the dynamics of my marriage to Charlie. So how could having a baby possibly change such a core component of my identity?

Little did I know.

MY MOMMY MOJO EXPERIENCE:
FROM MOJO TO *NOJO*

When I gave birth to our son, Rocky, I felt like a glowing warrior goddess.

In that moment, I was more feminine, powerful, and sensual than ever before. I felt more love than I could imagine—for our baby, my husband, myself—and even my own mother and father.

It felt magical, like I'd done what I was born to do. And I was so very happy.

But as the weeks passed and the newborn high subsided, the days and nights started blurring together. My energy fizzled out. I went from drowsy to exhausted to flat-out broken down from sleep deprivation. My breasts ached and leaked, and my brain felt fuzzy. I felt utterly unsexy, and totally alien in my own skin.

You see, before becoming a mom, I knew who I was: confident, sexy, and successful. I had built a career, married the love of my life, founded a flourishing business, penned my first book, appeared in national media, and led sexy seminars for celebrities. I went into motherhood on cloud nine, self-assured and fulfilled. But as happy as I was to welcome my boy into the world, I'd be lying if I didn't admit that becoming a mother also turned my whole life upside down.

When I became a mother, my core identity changed. I didn't know exactly who I was anymore. I was no longer *Dana, the founder of this, the writer of that* . . . Suddenly, I was Rocky's mommy. I didn't yet know myself as a mother, and it took some time to figure out who this new "me" really was. Motherhood wasn't just about learning how to care for a baby, but rather, a journey of learning how to love and accept the woman, wife, *and* mother I became when I entered parenthood.

Every decision I made suddenly took on new meaning. My emotions were different; my priorities changed. Past concerns and interests seemed trivial. My energy was both sky-high and completely shot at the same time. Not to mention my body felt like it belonged to someone else.

And along with these changes came a shift in my relationship to my partner.

We were madly in love with our baby and enamored with the creative process of family life. But it didn't take long before I began to feel a little disconnected from my husband. I was impatient, annoyed, and resentful that he went to work while I was stuck at home. We were so focused on becoming good parents, on not screwing up this massive responsibility, that we began to lose sight of our own relationship. Like most new parents, we were stumbling and struggling to fit romance and fun into our new life.

After a couple months of healing, I felt a deep, physical urge to return to sex with my man. Yes! There I was again! Well . . . *sort of.* Although the pain that lingered from childbirth had subsided and the return of my ability to orgasm reminded me of how much I enjoy having sex, that "deep, physical urge" was often fleeting. I was, like most moms, just too damn tired to get it on. I wasn't interested, and I felt as though my innate sexuality was on pause, indefinitely. In some moments, I would even think to myself, *I have a baby now—what do I need sex for anymore?*

How was it possible that I was both interested and totally *uninterested* in sex at the same time?

I must admit this confused me: I knew that sexual intimacy and pleasure were necessary components to the well-being of my own body and mind as well as for the health of my marriage, but, nevertheless, I resisted.

Though we slowly began to have sex again, we settled into the standard parent routine of one quickie per week. I wondered whether something that was once so pleasurable, natural, and exploratory for my husband and me would ever be the same again.

Every day, I woke up struggling to balance the roles of mother, professional, wife, lover and woman. *Where was the sparkling, sexy, turned on Dana I used to be? I had to find her. I had to wake her up! I had to discover who she could become in this next phase of womanhood...*

It just simply wasn't an option *not to.*

I changed out of my yoga pants and nursing bra and picked up my first book, *The Official Booty Parlor Mojo Makeover: Four Weeks to a Sexier You.* I dove back into the activities and practices, but this time, I looked at everything through a mother's eyes, with a new perspective. I was focused on finding fun, creative ways to solve the very real, very unglamorous challenges I was facing as a new mom.

Every day, I did *something* to reawaken my sexuality and rediscover my sensual confidence, reconnect with my post-baby body, and reignite the lust in my relationship.

With a lot of tweaking to accommodate my busy mama's schedule, I put a new spin on my original advice. I developed sensual self-care exercises to rebuild my body confidence, and communication tools to reduce the resentment I so often felt toward my husband in an effort to revitalize our romantic connection. I reinstated a regular self-pleasuring practice, learned how to carve out me-time, and made an effort to go wild with my girlfriends. I also gave myself permission to retool my professional desires to help shift my work/life balance. Of course, I invited my man to be a part of the great Mommy Mojo experiment, and swiftly transitioned us out of our quickie-only routine. And sure enough, I watched in wonder as my libido steadily began to rise. I felt as though I was bravely stepping into and embracing the new me—a sensual, turned-on, red-hot mama. I had committed to allowing my erotic energy to flow once again . . . and wow, did it ever pay off!

And to this very day, my Mommy Mojo practice still works like a charm. After thirteen years of marriage with two children in tow, I feel sexier, happier, and more confident and satisfied than ever before. The passion in my marriage continues to evolve and grow in ways I never could have imagined. My orgasms are bigger and better. Our communication in and out of the bedroom only continues to get stronger. And while motherhood is often trying and chaotic, and our relationship has had its fair share of ups and downs, there is something deep within me that is calm, centered, *and* turned on, knowing that I'm continuing to nurture the sexiest version of myself and fanning the flames of desire within my marriage. Moreover, I'm one hundred percent certain that I'm a better mother—with more patience, presence, sparkle and vitality—simply by feeling like the sexiest, most confident woman I can be.

Now it's both my mission and passion to help other mamas out there reclaim happiness, sexiness, and satisfaction in life and relationship. Because I fully believe the old saying is true: "If Mama ain't happy, ain't nobody happy!"

YOUR MOMMY MOJO MAKEOVER EXPERIENCE

I believe that as mothers, we have an amplified sensual power. We've experienced the most divine act possible: we created life. We keep other human beings alive. We've tapped into a primal feminine source, and because of it, we are smarter, we feel more, we love more, we're more tuned into our intuition and we can experience more pleasure. The potency of our sensual superpower drives us toward a sexier life and relationship. So this is a good thing: motherhood gives us more Mojo! We just have to fire it up.

So Mama, are you ready to get started?

Together, we'll explore twenty-eight tools and lessons that address all the Mommy Mojo Blocks you may be experiencing: feeling stuck in the Mom Zone, having a lazy libido, experiencing a loss of romantic connection, struggling with bedroom boredom, and even hating your own body—to name a few. I've been through all of it myself and I tried countless ways to get to the other side. But only the best tools made the cut into this book for you.

Throughout the process, you can expect to be challenged; to have fun, to laugh and cry—and to be pushed out of your comfort zone to increase the frequency and variety within your sex life. It doesn't matter how tired or busy you are, or how much you feel the sexiest days of your relationship are behind you. Leave your excuses at the door! You *can* cultivate your own vibrant, sexy, hot mama self-confidence, and create a smashing sex life with yourself and your partner!

By the time you finish this book, you'll feel more free, playful, and inspired as a mother, and more wholly satisfied, joyful, and empowered as a sensual woman within your relationship. You'll discover a renewed enthusiasm for sex, and experience intensified sexual satisfaction and intimacy with yourself and your lover. Others will take notice and want what you've got! You'll inspire other mamas simply by being the most confident, fired up version of yourself. You'll feel more loved, worshipped, and adored, and will have rekindled the romance you've longed for. You'll possess more authentic, raw desire for sex, and the energy to actually enjoy it. Most importantly, you'll rebirth elements of discovery and newness in your relationship, which often fade over time.

The beauty of this program is that whether you implement a lesson every day for twenty-eight days straight, or simply attempt one tool per week, you'll still see the results. The *Mommy Mojo Makeover* works best when you take consistent action and implement small but powerful changes on a regular basis. These shifts will eventually add up to make a huge difference in your life. But even when you're crunched for time, know that you can flip open to any page and you'll get something inspirational out of it.

Throughout our lives, and of course, our pregnancies, our Mommy Mojo continues to shift and evolve, contract and expand. It's my hope that you can always return to the *Mojo Makeover* for help and inspiration, and a little tune-up whenever you need it.

The Mommy Mojo Makeover is my love letter to you, Mama. It's my manifesto for sexy, modern motherhood and marriage. It's a pathway back to YOU, and forward into a relationship that thrills and turns you on.

So . . .

Stay open.

Do the work.

Make more time for yourself.

Learn to make love to yourself.

Be open in your communications.

Change your relationship patterns.

Lean on me and the sisters in our hot mama community.

(Find out how to connect at www.DanaBMyers.com)

And most of all—Have more orgasms, with yourself and your partner!!

This is your time to step into a more brilliant vision of motherhood, womanhood, and your relationship. Enjoy it, Mama!

Introducing The Mommy Mojo Makeover

BEFORE WE DIVE IN, take a moment to assess how you're feeling. Are you excited and intrigued, curious and raring to go, or maybe even a little skeptical? Don't worry, I'm going to ease you into this process. We'll begin by going over the Mommy Mojo Makeover plan so you can get a glimpse of just how we'll work together to reawaken your sensuality and rekindle your desire.

WHAT IS MOJO?

If we're going to be giving your Mojo a makeover, we should start by defining what Mojo means. Merriam-Webster defines mojo as "a magic spell, hex, or charm; broadly: magical power." (Yep, I'd have to agree on the *magical power* bit.) But I believe that Mojo is best defined as the feminine sexual spark that lies within every woman—it's a glow from the inside out. Mojo is your lust for life, love, sex, pleasure, and all the juicy possibilities that are available to all of us. It is your *sex*—your sexual attitude, your sexual drive, your personal sexual magnetism, and a reflection of how confident and free you feel to express yourself sexually. In other words, your Mojo is, in essence, the primordial expression of your *sex*.

Mommy Mojo is more than just confidence, it's *sexy* self-confidence integrated with the rich wisdom and experience of motherhood. It's your ability to know, embrace, and love your post-baby body, to know your desires and feel empowered to communicate them and to confidently prioritize yourself, your sensual satisfaction, and your intimate relationship with your partner—just as much as you prioritize your own children and well-being.

Learning to embrace your Mommy Mojo is about choosing love over resentment, sexiness over sexlessness, and self-care over self-neglect. It's about choosing to be sexually expressive instead of shut down. In empowering yourself to make these choices, you become more in tune with the wildness inside of you, falling in love—and hopefully lust!—with yourself and your spouse over and over again.

IS THIS *REALLY* FOR ME?

Having kids changes *everything*. If you're reading this book, it's likely that your marriage, partnership, or relationship has fallen into a sexual rut since you and your partner became parents. There's also a good chance that motherhood has left you feeling exhausted, overwhelmed, and disconnected from your body and your sensuality. Yet you still yearn to be turned on, and you long for that deep romantic, sexual connection you once had with your partner.

Whether you've got a six-month-old still suckling at your breasts or you're wrangling four-year-old twins at the park or you're picking up your kids from junior high, this book is for ALL moms. However, this book will be the most useful when you're fresh out of the "honeymoon phase" of parenting, when your baby has graduated to the

While I am a sexy lifestyle expert, I am *not* a doctor and the advice in this book is not medical. If you have medical questions about your health or hormones, please consult your family doctor or OB/GYN. If you are grappling with an intense challenge, such as the discovery of an affair or the emotional wounds of past sexual trauma, or if you think you may be experiencing postpartum depression, please seek the help of a professional therapist. You are not alone and do not need to suffer in silence. Please reach out for help!

♥ ♥ ♥

In this book, the distinctions of woman and man (as well as mother/father, mama/daddy, and the pronouns him and her) are used as a structure for talking about the experience of parenthood. Please know that this program will work for people of *all* genders and sexual orientations; any parent can use these tools and exercises to get their sexy Mojo back.

toddler zone. Your body has fully healed from your birth experience, you're (hopefully) sleeping again, you've honed in on a routine that works, and you've emerged from the "baby brain" fog. This is the perfect moment to dig in, discover, and develop the positive practices and habits that will reignite your sensual radiance and strengthen your relationship bond to give your sex life a much needed (and well-deserved) boost.

THE MOMMY MOJO MAKEOVER ACTION PLAN: HOW IT WORKS

The Mommy Mojo Makeover is comprised of twenty-eight actionable tools and lessons to empower you to reignite your Mojo. You'll rediscover your vibrant sensuality and reconnect to your post-baby body, and rekindle an erotic spark in your relationship.

You can read and use as many tools as you'd like whenever you have time, but you are encouraged to practice one tool each day. Each tool may contain a sexy shift in perspective to ponder, a journaling prompt, a self-love practice to explore, a communication exercise to try with your partner, or a sex assignment to get down and dirty with.

All the tools are designed to inspire you to conjure the innate sexiness that's inside of you, but has fallen asleep at the wheel since having kids. You'll learn to pay more attention to yourself and your needs, to reinvest in the romance in your relationship, and to enhance the frequency, variety, and pleasure in your sex life. The makeover process is freeing, feminine, and satisfying—but daring at times, too. This work requires dedication and a big step outside your comfort zone, and a true commitment to yourself and your partner.

If you're concerned about this process adding *more* pressure to your relationship, I encourage you to drop those doubts and fears immediately. The expectations we place on our relationship are already outrageously high. We expect one person to give us sizzling romance and familiar friendship at the same time. We want intense physical attraction *and* equality in our domestic duties. We hope that our core values are shared when it comes to parenting and money, and yet somehow along the way, we'd like to keep the mystery and intrigue alive in the bedroom.

Is it really possible to have all of this, *and* more? Yes! But it starts with YOU. Rekindling true desire comes from reconnecting with yourself first. This plan will challenge you to tap into the mastery of your own sexuality so that you can evolve into the fullest, juiciest, most empowered and satisfied experience of womanhood, motherhood, and partnership. Your partner will also get on board with you, so do keep in mind that you're not going through this alone. Here's what you can expect:

♥ **A Kick-Off Questionnaire:** You'll identify and explore your Mommy Mojo Blocks, those common obstacles that get in the way of your personal satisfaction, sexual desire, and romantic connection. You'll then set exciting and achievable goals for your journey to change, grow, and rediscover the innate sexiness that's inside of you.

♥ **Twenty-Eight Tools, Lessons, and Exercises:** These are designed to help you reconnect to your Mojo. Each tool builds upon the next to lovingly coax out an inspired and empowered sensuality and organically heighten your desire. You'll learn how to *Reboot Your Body Confidence*, experience the pleasure of a *Solo Session*, create time to *Go Wild with Your Mom Tribe*, be challenged to *Reduce the Resentment* in your relationship, and even discover your *Sexual Superpowers*. And there's *plenty* more.

You can follow the tools in order—one every day for twenty-eight days—to experience a complete sensual transformation and romance rehab in just four weeks. Now, because time is *always* an issue for us busy mamas, you can also try implementing just one to three tools per week. You could also just open the book to any page whenever you like for a hit of sexy inspiration, especially when you have only five minutes to spare. The idea behind this is really to create your own experience.

♥ **The Sexy Sessions:** There are eight sexy experiences designed to jumpstart your sexual chemistry, shake up bedroom boredom, encourage you to explore creative and different pathways to your pleasure, and invigorate you as a sensual woman and couple. The Sexy Sessions are practices that inspire increased frequency, variety, and satisfaction in your sex life. You might imagine them as a ladder to climb toward reinstating your sexual chemistry and satisfaction: eight steps to ascend, all leading toward a revived, passionate sex life. But beyond the immediate surge of sexual activity the Sessions inspire, this practice is a route to reestablishing honest sexual communication, deeper emotional intimacy and a juicier romantic connection with your partner.

The Sexy Sessions are:

1. The Solo Session
2. The Quickie
3. The Long Love Engagement
4. The BJ
5. Fantasy Fun
6. Receiving Pleasure
7. Playing Together
8. Spontaneous Sex

If you're doing your makeover as a four-week program, **you'll explore two Sexy Sessions each week**. Many moms tell me their sexual frequency since having kids has been reduced to once every seven to ten days. The Sexy Sessions ask that you commit to boosting that number in order to shift your relationship out of its rut and into new territory. Don't worry, it doesn't have to be *amazing* sex every single time, so you can take that pressure off yourself right away. The goal of having two Sessions per week is to help you two create a sense of playfulness and exploration within your sex life again. When you're having sex more often, you're making space for a variety of "sexual energies" to arise between you—one Session might be heated, the next time tender, a few days later dirty and raw, and then vulnerable, loving, and spiritual. Tasting all those "flavors" together is *fun*, adds variety back into your relationship, and helps you remember just how amusing and connective sex can be. And if you're only having sex once a week, there's just not enough opportunity to do that.

♥ **Real-World Advice:** Along the way, you'll be encouraged by true stories from my own journey in motherhood, as well as anecdotes from other real women just like you: brave, unique mamas who've completed their own Mojo Makeover journeys in my workshops or through one-on-one coaching sessions with me.

♥ **A Maintenance Plan:** Hitting a goal is awesome, but staying there is even sweeter. When you've explored all twenty-eight tools, it's important to continue to practice them; you don't want to leave your Mojo high and dry. With the Mommy Mojo Maintenance Plan, you'll be equipped with the tips, tricks, and inspiration you need to keep your sexy mama revolution going indefinitely.

THE TOOLS FOR YOUR MAKEOVER

Before you start exercising your Mojo muscles, it's important that you prep for your journey. Here are a few things you'll need as you prepare to start your makeover:

TIME—I know you are a busy mama with a busy schedule, and the time you have to devote to this process is limited. However, you are just as important as everything else you *have* to do in your life. It's time to *make time* for yourself and your sex life, to make your pleasure a priority again—or perhaps for the first time in your life!

Not all the tools in this book require the same amount of time. Some ask that you "steal" ten minutes of alone time, while others insist that you block out several hours to indulge in a full-on sensual experiment with your partner. On other days, you might read a lesson and do some journaling while cheering on your kid during an after-school activity. To create more time, take a good look at your day: Can you put the kids to bed thirty minutes earlier to give you extra grown-up time with your spouse? Can you reduce the time you spend scrolling on Facebook in order to fit in your Sexy Mama Meditation? Can you set your alarm for fifteen minutes earlier than usual to practice your sensual self-care rituals? What can you delegate to someone else in order to squeeze in an extra hour on that afternoon date you've planned? Can you say no more often, to more things, so that you feel less overcommitted and have more energy for yourself and for sex?

I know the juggle is real for all of us mamas, especially on the domestic front, so choose your battles wisely to make more time for your makeover. Choose what you can live with (like unmade beds) and what will drive you crazy (like dirty bathrooms). If you want to create more time for this experience, you're going to have to loosen your grip on your quest for domestic perfection. The dishes can wait!

SLEEP—You need sleep to feel like a human, and you need to feel like a human again to embark on this sexy adventure! So, if you are in the thick of newborn babydom, breastfeeding, and excruciating sleep deprivation, I implore you: PLEASE DON'T START THIS MAKEOVER YET! Be sure you're sleeping through the night—or, at least, getting a decent chunk of uninterrupted sleep—before attempting to bring your Mojo back.

Also, please give yourself permission to nap as much as you need to, no matter what stage of motherhood you're in. Even now, with both my kids sleeping through the night, I try to take a twenty-minute power nap several times a week. A short nap could give you the extra energy you need to rally for the Session of Fantasy Fun you penciled in and the Mommy Pop-Out you so deserve.

HELP—If you don't do this already (or don't do it enough), I encourage you to get in the babysitting game, and fast. Calling in for backup will give you the time and space you need to decompress from being Supermom, and to reconnect with yourself as a woman and partner. A babysitter is going to give you the much-needed me-time you truly deserve as part of this process. Yes, you are a fantastic mother—but you don't have to be there 24/7. Call your parents, in-laws, neighbors, best friends, nannies, or high-school babysitter, and book some babysitting hours as part of your makeover process. If your budget is tight, dig deep to see what you can shuffle around. For instance, how many lattes would you give up in order to book a date night sitter?

ATTITUDE—A truly satisfying sex life requires education, communication, commitment, and confidence. It asks that you shift your attitude from seeing sex as a chore, to something pleasurable that you have the privilege of doing with the partner you love. If you're reading this book, you're already pretty damned committed to improving your intimate connection with your spouse. So before you begin, take a moment to sit with your love and commit to following these four principles as you take on the Sexy Sessions and more within this program. Discuss and explore what they mean to you and the work you're doing together:

♥ **Priority**

By reading this book and committing to the Sexy Sessions together, you're both choosing to make your sex life a PRIORITY. What is it going to take, however, to keep it a priority as the weeks and months go by? Scheduling time for intimate conversations outside the bedroom? Agreeing to only work late only twice a week? Putting down your phones when you're in the bedroom together? Or, perhaps you need to create a more efficient bedtime routine for the kids, so you get two full hours of togetherness in the evenings? Remember: Couples who make their sex lives a priority wind up with epic sex lives!

♥ Planning

There's no doubt that planning out your Sexy Sessions will give you both a positive framework to make improvements in your sex life. Yes, this means sitting down at the start of each week and actually scheduling in when you'll try out each of the Sessions! If you're concerned that planning will make sex feel too staged, or that it takes the romance out of it, consider how can you make the planning more fun? Can you think of it as an invitation to experience pleasure together instead of a scheduled task? Can you sketch out your Sexy Sessions together as an out-of-the-bedroom ritual, over dinner with cocktails and music? Remember: Planning keeps your sex life active, frequent, and in a consistent rhythm, which opens the door for more spontaneous sex to emerge!

♥ Flexibility

We all know the saying about the best laid plans, right? Planning is great, but we all know that life throws curveballs into our schedules, meaning that Sunday night's Session might get pushed back due to a family emergency. Your child might come down with the flu on the night you've planned a Playtime Session, or a project keeps you or your spouse at the office until midnight. How can you continue to prioritize and incorporate planning into your sex life, while staying flexible and open to integrating more spontaneous sex in your relationship? It might be as easy as agreeing that a Long Love Engagement becomes a Quickie, or that you'll try to fit in two Sessions over a ten-day span, instead of seven.

♥ Follow-Through

For the flexibility part to work, you both have to commit to following through with the work to maintain your trust. If your spouse is frequently disappointed because you keep finding reasons to skip out on your Sessions, it'll be hard for him to trust that you're committed to the makeover process. Following through on your Sessions will lead to less disappointment and pressure that could be felt from you both. This will help you feel that your needs are being met, allowing for more compassion to permeate your intimate connection.

Sex Toys

Whether you're currently a vibrator expert or a total beginner, sex toys and sensual accessories can play a very important role in your Mojo Makeover, by aiding in more frequent and legendary orgasms. You will be asked to self-pleasure on a weekly basis, so if you've already got a treasured tool to get you where you want to go, fantastic! If you're in need of one, then you'll need to treat yourself; if you are self-conscious about going into an adult store, there are plenty of websites that will deliver a toy quickly and discreetly to your front door.

Your Journal

I recommend you have a journal handy to document your thoughts and experiences, your O-Notes, and other feedback on your sexy communication exercises. Often, you are the best person to help you understand what you're feeling, so notes in your own voice will be helpful.

DITCHING THE "I CAN'T" EXCUSES

Now that you're clearer about your Mommy Mojo Makeover path, it may have raised some questions—or, some resistance. Let's look at the most common excuses, obstacles, and resistance I frequently encounter at the onset of a mama's makeover:

I'm too busy.

Aren't all mamas? Like I said above, I know you have a busy multitasking life, and that's exactly why you should stick with the program. It's your turn to focus on you now! This program can actually help you get more creative with how you spend your time and even discover how to create more of it for yourself.

That seems like A LOT of sex!

Here's the thing: sex begets sex. When you have some, it's easier to have (and want) more. It's just like working out—once you start, you remember how good it feels and it's easier to get yourself to the gym. The Sexy Sessions are the same: One sexual interaction feels good and inspires you to show up for the next. The hotter the Sessions become, the more enthusiasm you'll organically feel to keep showing up!

But isn't planning sex a drag?

It all depends on how you look at it. Of course, many couples miss the spontaneous sex they enjoyed before having kids. But if we didn't plan it, most couples with kids probably wouldn't have it. With the variety included in the Sexy Sessions, you'll discover that scheduled sex can be just as steamy as getting hot and heavy on a whim. Planning the Sessions isn't about adding more pressure to your already chaotic life or putting a stringent quota on your sex life. It's about getting you into a fresh sexual routine that's focused on frequency, variety, and satisfaction. And the truth is that you need to have a fair amount of scheduled sex in order for the opportunity of spontaneous sex to organically arise again.

Still, I'm not totally comfortable with my post-baby body . . .

Many mamas resist self-pleasuring or fully expressing themselves in the bedroom because they're uncomfortable with their post-baby bodies and the extra weight they're carrying. Please Mama, don't deny yourself pleasure because of a few extra pounds or some stretch marks! This book will show you how to give yourself the permission to own your body—as it is, right now—and to love yourself in your own skin.

Won't this divert my attention away from my kids?

Yes, and gloriously so! Many of us moms claim that our children are our entire world, and this is of course true in our hearts. But as parents, we also need to nurture ourselves as individuals, and our sensuality is a HUGE part of that. Don't try to convince yourself that your kids can't be without you or that you can't be without them. Scoring more me-time and more we-time with your spouse will actually *benefit* your children. Having a happier, more confident mama who feels empowered in her own sexuality and deserving of pleasure will set a powerful example for your children.

My past gets in the way of my sexual liberation.

I know that sexual trauma, guilt, and shame can rob you of your Mojo, increase your stress toward sex, decrease your self-esteem, and cause you to shut down. If your own sexual past is holding you back, I encourage you to have compassion for yourself and begin healing. This may mean talking through your feelings with your partner, best friend, or a therapist, or offering up deep forgiveness for yourself and others. When you avoid processing any shame or guilt you may be feeling, you only create more of the same, which disconnects you from your sexuality. Through self-compassion, you can begin to release your pain and embrace the healthy, pleasure-filled sex life and confidence you deserve.

Lastly, ask yourself whether there are any other obstacles that could stand in your way of bringing back your Mojo. Take a moment to write down anything that may come to mind in your journal, and then get ready to uncover what's possible for you as a woman, a wife, and a mother.

Exploring Mojo Blocks And Setting Goals For Your Transformation

MOTHERHOOD IS PART BLISS, part chaos; equally rewarding as it is stifling. Parenting with a partner can be the most beautiful bonding experience, but it can also be a breeding ground for resentment, romantic disconnect, and unsatisfying sex.

No matter how many kids you have or how long you've been with your spouse, I've found that most moms encounter a few common obstacles as they seek out the sexiest, most satisfying expression of their self-confidence and relationship. Whether you know these blocks as *mojo malfunctions, mommy problems,* or *mommy pains,* it makes no difference. They've drained you of desire, lowered your self-esteem, and left you wondering if passion will ever return to your partnership.

Before we start whipping your Mommy Mojo into shape, let's discover your blocks. Let's fearlessly shed some light on what's been holding you back from being the amazingly alluring and inspired woman, mother, and partner you're meant to be.

Mommy Blocks

Through my constant sex chatter with moms at my workshops (and playdates, too), I began to notice eight common themes. As you read through each one I've listed below, notice whether you knowingly nodded along in agreement, shouting *YES, that's me*! Or, maybe there was only one that really stood out to you as a red flag. Consider these as wake-up calls, and then keep them in mind as you move through the tools in the book. The solutions will start to reveal themselves as you make your way through the process. (After each Mommy Mojo Block, there are journaling questions for you to answer.)

Every time you recognize a challenge in your life as a potential Mommy Mojo Block, try freewriting your responses—and be as specific as possible. These are the areas that need the most love and attention during your twenty-eight-day transformation, so being honest and authentic is the *most* important thing you can do.

THE EIGHT BIGGEST MOMMY MOJO BLOCKS

1. The Mom Zone

You have a super-busy life balancing the many responsibilities of motherhood. Between schoolwork and activities, cooking dinner and tending to your kids' every need, the pressure to parent perfectly is burning you out. Whenever you see your friends (probably on a play-date), your conversations revolve around kids and are constantly interrupted by them. Sometimes you feel overwhelmed by the demands of motherhood and that you're lacking the personal freedom you desire. You might even feel bored to tears with your domestic load, and left wondering where the real you went. Sex has fallen low on your priority list, which is not that surprising considering how much energy you give to your kids. Since you don't have the energy to nurture the sexy woman within, you feel stuck in the Mom Zone.

Ask yourself the following questions:
- ♥ *What contributes to you getting stuck in the Mom Zone?*
- ♥ *How do you feel when you notice yourself in the Mom Zone—physically and emotionally?*
- ♥ *If you're able to pull yourself out of the Mom Zone every now and again, what have you noticed helps you do it?*

To bust through this block, pay attention to the following Tools:

Go Wild with Your Mom Tribe

Infuse Every Day with Sexy Stimulation

Own Your Sexual Superpower

2. Low Libido

Since becoming a mother, your desire has been on a slow and steady decline. From hormonal shifts to sleep deprivation, chronic stress, and physical exhaustion, your sexual appetite has waned. It's also possible that after a long day of the kids hanging from your every limb, you're "all touched out" and just want to be left alone once they're asleep! Motherhood requires being 100 percent "on" all the time, and so you're always thinking about the safety, well-being, and development of your little creatures. This constant mental multitasking—and likely a lack of self-care—leaves you feeling physically and mentally drained, and sexually uninspired. It's no wonder you're too tired to make love after the kids are in bed.

Ask yourself the following questions:
- ♥ *How has motherhood—and all its mental and physical exhaustion—affected your libido?*
- ♥ *Is your spouse emotionally supportive when you open up about your*

lack of desire? Is he open to working together to find solutions for you to feel less exhausted and to replenish yourself sensually?

♥ *Are you currently using any form of birth control that may be contributing to your lack of libido?*

To bust through this block, pay attention to the following Tools:

The Solo Session: A Sexy Session

Create a Sexy Self-Care Strategy

Take Time to Meditate

3. Body Confidence

Some moms feel just as amazing as they did pre-baby, regardless of whether their bodies changed, but many more moms view their body in a very different way post-baby. If you're one of those moms, you may feel depressed about your appearance, or even hate how you look. Your inner vixen doesn't give you a wink when you look in the mirror anymore. Maybe you've started to reject your spouse's compliments, or you turn off the lights during sex to hide your body. You might find yourself talking trash about your thighs, tush, or tummy. There's never enough time to exercise the way you like or get your favorite beauty and self-care treatments, all of which leaves you feeling less than thrilled with your post-baby body.

Ask yourself the following questions:

♥ *What are the most pervasive thoughts you have about your body?*

♥ *Do you go out of your way to hide your body from your partner, yourself, the world? If so, how?*

♥ *When was the last time you looked in the mirror and appreciated what you saw?*

To bust through this block, pay attention to the following Tools:

    Reboot Your Body Confidence

    Dance to Ignite Your Sensuality

    Receiving Pleasure: A Sexy Session

4. Time

You're short on it. Short on me-time. Short on kid-free time with your spouse. Short on time to do what you love and to see your girlfriends. You feel like you're barely getting through your to-do list, let alone finding a moment to decompress and leisurely think about sensual things or get busy in the bedroom. The carefree bonding time you once shared as a couple has winnowed away to nearly nothing. Not only are you desperately short on precious together time, you and your spouse may be prioritizing time in different ways—causing your busy schedules to feel out of sync and driving a wedge between you.

Ask yourself the following questions:

♥ *What would you do if you had more free time every week?*

♥ *How does your lack of time affect your dynamic with your partner?*

♥ *What is your ideal working balance between me-time and we-time?*

To bust through this block, pay attention to the following Tools:

    The Mommy Pop-Out

    Bring Back that Lovin' Feeling

    Make Date Night a Priority

5. Identity Crisis

There is a very real identity crisis that happens when you become a mother—and no one seemed to warn you about it! Perhaps you were once a social butterfly, with seemingly unlimited time and freedom to explore restaurants, hang out with friends, or take trips. Maybe you were an ultra-productive rock star at work, and then slipped on sexy heels and went salsa dancing at night. You defined yourself by your accomplishments, your passions, your talents. And then you became a mom: "So-and-so's mom." Perhaps you chose to take a break from work to raise them. And then you question, *Am I just a mom now?* And, *Am I a good enough mom?* And perhaps the biggest one of all, *Why aren't I having more fun with this?!* The sudden lack of freedom and the enormous responsibility of caring for a child is a big deal, and it can make you feel like you've lost yourself. You might sometimes wonder: *Where is the fun, social, sensual woman I used to be?*

Ask yourself the following questions:
- ♥ *In what ways do you feel like a different version of yourself than before you had kids?*
- ♥ *What do you miss about your pre-kids self?*
- ♥ *What has shocked you most about the way you define yourself since becoming a mom?*

To bust through this block, pay attention to the following Tools:
Stop Trying to Be Perfect
Choose Fun over Obligation
Do What You Desire

6. Romantic Disconnect
When you brought your baby home, you immersed yourselves in the blissful experience of *becoming parents*. You swore that having kids wouldn't change your relationship, but it did anyway. You became

incredible partners in parenting, and maybe even better friends than you thought possible, but the sex went from hot to obligatory—and the desire and erotic tension you once had for each other began to fizzle out. The steadiness and routine that helps family life run so smoothly has zapped all spontaneity, flirtation, and adventure. Your conversations with your partner are now mostly about the kids, and your once-a-week date nights have turned into once-a-month outings where you're home by nine. Perhaps you're even feeling a genuine loss of sexual attraction, and worry he feels the same. The loss of romantic connection is one of the most gut-wrenching and pervasive pains of motherhood!

Ask yourself the following questions:
- ♥ *What do you miss most about your romantic connection?*
- ♥ *What do you think your partner misses most about your romance?*
- ♥ *How have you and your spouse talked about your current disconnect, if at all?*

To bust through this block, pay attention to the following Tools:

Let's Talk about Sex, Baby

The Long Love Engagement, a Sexy Session

Make Date Night a Priority

7. Resentment

Many moms have shared with me that they resent their spouse because they feel unsupported. Moms tend to take on more of the childcare and domestic responsibilities, and can feel like we're just not getting enough help, appreciation, or acknowledgment. Working moms, SAHMs, ultramodern progressive moms, hippie moms, it doesn't matter: moms just take on more. But the resentment creeps in when he rarely-to-never takes charge of the kids' activities. Or when he leaves for the gym, hangs out with friends, or works on a passion project without considering family responsibilities. It seems like you're always the one who has to secure childcare while you squeeze in your "other" life (work, hobbies, friends, self-care, etc.) between errands and playdates. Maybe he's the breadwinner and feels entitled to relax after his workday, while yours just keeps going. Nothing kills the desire for intimate, connected sex like simmering resentment; when it goes unchecked, it can lead to intense hurt and anger, which can (surprise!) result in less sex.

Ask yourself the following questions:
- ♥ *When do you feel resentment toward your partner creep up?*
- ♥ *What do you wish you and/or your partner would do differently to lessen the resentment you feel?*
- ♥ *Do you think your partner feels resentment toward you? If so, what about?*

To bust through this block, pay attention to the following Tools:
Reduce the Resentment
Learn to Love Daddy Style
Playing Together, a Sexy Session

8. Unsatisfying Sex

There was probably a time in the not-so-distant past when you couldn't imagine using "bedroom" and "boring" in the same sentence. In the pre-baby phase of your relationship, your sex life was hot, heavy, passionate . . . and you expected it to be that way forever. But now, your lovemaking has slowed down to a predictable, uninspiring once-a-week affair: you know exactly what's coming because it's always the same. Worse, your sex drives often feel way out of sync: maybe he wants more, you want less—and you might even feel pressure from him because of it and struggle to turn off your brain and let go during the act. Or maybe you both are stuck in a cycle of sexual fatigue from the relentless emotional and physical stresses of parenting. You're both spending your energy just getting through another day, and little is left over for feeling turned on together.

Ask yourself the following questions:

♥   *What do you miss most about your pre-parenthood sex life?*

♥   *How has your sex drive changed since becoming a mom?*

♥   *What do you wish you could say to your spouse about your current sex life?*

To bust through this block, pay attention to the following Tools:

Let's Talk about Sex, Baby

Inspire Desire

Fantasy Fun, A Sexy Session

What other Mommy Mojo Blocks are you experiencing?

Please take a moment to express any other mommy blocks you're experiencing. There truly is no right or wrong problem, and no single way to feel. If something has been nagging at you and it wasn't recognized above, describe it below:

_____

_____

_____

_____

_____

Check-In!

Now that you've completed the questions, take a few moments to decompress. It's likely that a lot of feelings came up as you read through the Mommy Mojo Blocks. Maybe you felt a sense of sadness or a surge of resentment. Take a few minutes to acknowledge what you're feeling, and then get excited for what's next: your transformation action plan.

ACTION PLAN:
SETTING GOALS FOR YOUR TRANSFORMATION

Truth: You are in charge of your own happiness, freedom, and satisfaction. And I believe that YOU set the tone for your relationship and sex life. If you are happy and possess a sense of freedom as a woman and mother, your relationship will feel alive and exciting. If you are giving yourself sensual pleasure, you will crave more pleasure from your partner. But if you are annoyed and angry and resentful all the time, then your relationship will reflect that. (Of course, it takes two to tango. It's critical that your partner sets goals for making positive changes alongside you as part of this process.)

No matter how many of the Mommy Mojo Blocks you identified with, know that you can be an awesome mom and a sexy, turned-on woman while living in the relationship of your dreams. It's your right! And while it takes some hard work, planning, and flexibility, you don't actually need to sacrifice a thing.

As you begin this transformational journey, let's set an intention and commitment for your experience—this work requires it. You might say your intention quietly to yourself or out loud. Write it down. Tell your partner. Share it with a friend. Invite them to support you as you begin.

To get started, here are some examples of intention statements. Circle the ones you'd like to call your own, and write anything additional in your journal.

♥ I want to rediscover a heightened enthusiasm for sex and an expanded desire and confidence to talk about sex with my partner.

♥ I want to rekindle the elements of discovery, newness, and adventure that have faded in my relationship.

♥ I want more me-time.

♥ I want to feel more supported by my husband, and I want more help.

♥ I want to boost my libido.

♥ I want to love my body.

♥ I want to feel and emanate more sensual energy in my daily life.

♥ I want to let go of my guilt and shame and give myself the permission sexually to explore pleasure—without feeling burdened.

♥ I want to initiate sex again.

♥ I want to respond with a more authentic *yes* when my partner initiates.

♥ I want more romance from and with my husband.

♥ I want to have more orgasms.

♥ I want more variety in my sex life. I want to try new things!

♥ I want to stop playing the blame game and be a team again.

♥ I want to stop over-parenting and make more space for me, and for us.

♥ I want to be less stressed so I can feel sexier and more relaxed.

♥ I want to communicate more effectively with my spouse, in and out of the bedroom.

♥ I want more childcare so I can have more me-time.

Okay, Mama! You've done a lot of work already, and we've only just begun. By acknowledging your Mojo Blocks, you may have already had a few a-ha moments about what you'd like to accomplish during your makeover. Keep all of this in mind as we venture forward.

IT'S TIME TO GET STARTED . . .

Are you ready to reawaken your Mojo and create sexual enthusiasm for your relationship? You are more than a mother; you are a radiant woman capable of experiencing great pleasure, and lighting up the room with your lust for life and fully embodied confidence. It's time to remember just how hot you are!

. . . .

PART ONE

Wake Up Your Mojo

. . . .

Reboot Your Body Confidence

LET'S DIVE RIGHT IN and tackle one of the biggest Mommy Mojo zappers of all: *Negative Body Banter*. It's that self-destructive mental chatter we inflict upon ourselves whenever we're down on our bodies and our beauty—and worse, sometimes we're not even aware that we're doing it. It's time for you to call yourself out on this nasty habit and take a huge step toward embracing your sexiness at *every* shape and size. (Cellulite, post-baby bellies, and imperfect breasts, beware: I'm coming at you with radical self-love!)

Full disclosure: I wasn't always teeming with Mommy Mojo. About a year after I'd given birth to my baby girl, I noticed my three-year-old son was repeatedly pinching his tummy. I observed him for a day or two, and then asked him how his tummy was feeling and why was he squeezing himself like that. He said, "Mommy, I saw you doing it."

Oh, crap. Yes, he did.

The real truth is that my tummy had become a "problem area" after my daughter was delivered via C-section. The painful recovery I endured meant that I couldn't exercise as soon or as much as I wanted to. But in hindsight I can also admit that I just wasn't as motivated anymore now that I had two little ones to look after.

Until that point I'd never really had a stubborn layer of fat around my middle. I had *thought* I was being patient and loving with myself about it, but the negative self-talk toward my tummy was slowly growing louder and manifesting in the ways I touched my body. My son was right—I *was* unconsciously poking and prodding my belly rolls. I silently berated myself, with my inner thoughts nagging me to the core: *What IS this? It's disgusting! How did Jess get a flat belly so soon after her second kid? This is it, Dana. You'll never have a hot body again.*

Seriously . . . what the hell? Here I was, leading workshops for the moms in my community about Sexy Self-Love and total body confidence and yet, I was serving myself an unhealthy dose of smack talk on the daily. I felt like a fraud. I was upset that I was being cruel to myself and worse, for doing it unconsciously in front of my kids.

My son's mimicking behavior sounded a wake-up call to drop the body shaming and get back on track with my practice of Sexy Self-Love, a philosophy I'd adhered to since my early twenties.

And so, the self-love affirmations began: *My tummy is healthy, supple, and gorgeous. My belly birthed two insanely delicious babies. There is strength and softness in my middle. I honor the power AND the pudge!* For me, the key to success with these affirmations was putting my hands on my belly and making deep eye contact with myself in the mirror. I was creating a romance with myself, whispering sweet compliments to myself as I touched myself up. (And yes, sometimes I cringed/laughed while I said these things to myself, too.)

I caressed my belly throughout the day: at the office and the grocery store, at home and everywhere else. I bared my midriff at hot yoga, and challenged myself to stare at my belly's reflection in the mirror at the studio with softness, love, and pride instead of judgment and disgust. Standing there in only my sports bra and leggings took a whole lot of confidence, and that in itself felt like a turn-on—a sizzling reconnection to the real me. I felt like myself again, and the hatred I'd directed toward my midsection soon faded away. I was celebrating—instead of bashing—that fleshy jiggle in my middle.

Another story about a girlfriend illuminates just how pervasive negative self-talk about our bodies can be. Not long after my own reckoning, a dear friend sent me an email sharing an exchange she'd had with her husband. They were heading out for a date and he'd said to her, "Wow! You look great in that dress!" Without missing a beat, she said, "Really? Ugh, I feel gross. I can't lose those last five pounds." Her husband's face dropped in disappointment—and so did hers, with the realization that her negativity was on full display in front of her children, who were standing in the same room.

Mamas, this language is gross . . . and just plain dangerous! Whether you're the only one hearing it, or it slips out of your mouth in front of your husband and kids, it has *got* to stop. The way my friend reacted squandered any chances of feeling like a hot and happy mama. She rejected a compliment from her loving husband, which hurt his feelings since he genuinely thought she looked stunning. In doing so, she denied herself pleasure by basking in the adoration he so freely dished out to her. She also crushed an opportunity to return the compliment, which could have sparked flirtation just as they were heading out for a fun, romantic evening. All this before we even got to the impact her negative message may have had on her kids.

Time to Make a Change

I believe that every mother has a story like this. It's no surprise: Our bodies change so dramatically throughout the experience of motherhood. We expand, we shrink, and then we do it all over again for another baby. We are literal shape-shifters. But instead of stepping into our power as life-givers and making peace with our miraculous bodies, we often end up feeling just, well, unsexy. We get caught in the grips of Negative Body Banter.

Aside from the obvious, there are many harmful implications of Negative Body Banter. You feel bad about yourself, sure, but you're also holding yourself back in the bedroom! Your negative self-talk keeps you from being utterly sexually free with your lover. It distracts you from being fully present in the moment and from losing yourself in sensual abandon. How do you expect to have great sex if you're self-conscious about how deflated your breasts look? It's nearly impossible to welcome your spouse's sensual adoration if you don't feel you deserve it based on the size of your thighs. To have great sex with the one you love means you've got to drop the body shaming and become present in the body that is yours *today* and every day.

As moms—as *women*—our shape is *always* changing. That's a given, so why do we give our weight so much weight? Why do we give our lumps and bumps so much power over how gorgeous, sexy, and confident we *should* feel about ourselves?

. . . .

Twenty pounds up, or ten pounds down, it's in your power
to rewrite the conversation you have
with yourself, *about* yourself!

. . . .

It's time to embrace your mommy body as a beautiful, remarkable, sensual miracle, deserving of adoration and positive sexual attention. That includes your birth battle scars, sagging breasts, stretch marks, extra roundness, and whatever other perceived flaws you're attached to. What matters most is that YOU believe you're beautiful, strong, and *hot damn sexy*. Because if you don't feel this way about yourself, how do you expect anyone else to? Also, if you don't learn to feel comfortable with your post-baby body, it's hard to want to be touched by your partner.

Empower yourself! Your body is begging for your love, and craving your positive attention. So, leave the Negative Body Banter behind for good and start feeling like the sexiest, most confident version of yourself. Follow these steps to stop the smack talk and set your confidence on fire—both in and out of the bedroom!

THE TOOL:
TRANSFORM NEGATIVE BODY BANTER INTO SEXY SELF-LOVE AFFIRMATIONS

Step 1: Think of the awful things you say to yourself about yourself.

Stand in front of the mirror and say it all out loud. Don't hold back, no matter how terrible your own words make you feel. Notice which body part or physical attribute takes the worst beating. Take a moment to write down those terrible thoughts, or even better, record yourself saying them on your phone. The challenge: try to remain impartial as you judge yourself.

Step 2: Flip those negatives around to say something loving instead.

Choose the harshest piece of Negative Body Banter and transform it into a positive, loving affirmation. Better yet, say something sexy! The goal is not to try and erase the effects of maternity from our bodies, but to seek to discover and acknowledge the *new* sexiness that emerges from within our experience of motherhood instead. Once you've gotten the hang of it, record yourself again on your phone. You may feel silly at first, but that's totally normal. It won't be long before this exercise makes you feel really good.

Here are a few examples:

NEGATIVE BODY BANTER	SEXY SELF-LOVE AFFIRMATION
My thighs and ass are gigantic.	I love my juicy buns and curvy legs as they are—I'm *gorgeous and strong*.
My boobs are deflated.	My breasts are sweet, petite, and still hot after nursing all these babies.
My ass is SO dimpled.	My tush is feminine, sexy, and worthy of being adored!
You're fat.	I love you. I really, *really*, love you.
My belly is sagging and covered in stretch marks.	My belly is a hot miracle. If I can grow a baby, I can do anything!
I'm embarrassed how I look "down there" after giving birth. My vagina is just not the same!	My pussy is sensual and magical . . . capable of creating life *and* receiving so much pleasure.
I don't want him to see me naked.	I own this new body with confidence and want to show it and share it with pride.

NOW, IT'S YOUR TURN! ADD YOUR OWN TRANSFORMED THOUGHTS HERE:

NEGATIVE BODY BANTER	SEXY SELF-LOVE AFFIRMATION

Step 3: Embody Your Words.

This part is important, *especially* if you have a habit of poking and pinching the bits you hate—or doing everything in your power to avoid looking at or touching them at all. Stand in front of the mirror with your hands on your body, right on the part you've negatively focused on. Give it a rub, a shake, a wiggle, a loving caress, a happy dance, a sexy swerve—all while you're saying your Sexy Self-Love Affirmation aloud.

Combining the verbal and physical elements of this exercise is the key to boosting your confidence and learning to love your body more than you ever thought possible.

Step 4: Practice, Practice, *Practice!*

Make this a daily practice: transform your words and actions whenever that nasty inner voice starts to attack. If you get stuck, listen to your recordings to remind you that transforming self-hatred into self-love is totally possible and easier than you think. Bonus: Take pictures or a video of yourself doing this self-love ritual to refer back to whenever you need a boost.

Step 5: Share Your Wisdom with a Mom in Need.

After you've turned your Negative Body Banter around, call a mom friend and tell her about it. Sharing is a beautiful way to reinforce your own self-love practice and help the other moms in your life to do the same. Here are some talking points:

♥ Share the specifics of your Negative Body Banter. You'll be amazed and relieved to discover how totally *not alone* you were in it.

♥ Share how you transformed it into a Sexy Self-Love Affirmation.

♥ Share how you touched your body during the exercise, and how it felt (good, bad, inspiring, awkward, etc.).

♥ Then, tell her how great you felt afterward!

If she's ready and willing to be guided through this process with you, share the tools and insight to help put a stop to her inner critic in its tracks. It feels pretty great when you can help a friend feel amazing about herself, too.

Now that the practice of getting real about body shaming has opened your eyes, I hope you feel empowered to love your body fully and completely with a renewed sense of confidence. But let's get real for a moment: decades of body hatred and negative self-talk is not necessarily going to vanish in an instant. *But it's a start.* And much like yoga, *it's a practice.* By simply initiating a nicer conversation with your body every time that gnarly inner voice begins to attack your tush, tummy, and thighs, you can start to move toward the sensual body freedom you deserve. By sprinkling a few tiny doses of this sexy, self-loving goodness into your soul each day, you *will* start to change the way you see and treat yourself. Do this for yourself! (But do it to set a powerful body-positive example for your kids too.) Cultivating body confidence through Sexy Self-Love Affirmations is the first major step to taking back your Mommy Mojo.

The Solo Session A Sexy Session

I'LL BE HONEST WITH YOU: I *just* masturbated. Right before I wrote this chapter, I gave myself a deep, cleansing, vibrating, body-shaking orgasm. I turned on some tunes and rolled around in the soft sheets on my bed. I danced with my sex toy like it was my lover. I moaned, breathed, and swayed as I played myself like an instrument. I stretched my pleasure until I couldn't hold back, and then I watched myself in the mirror as I came. It was sexy—and it was spiritual. It was affirming, animalistic, joyful and tender all at once.

Before that, I'd been sitting in my home office staring blankly at my computer screen, wondering how I was going to write this chapter. I began to sweat; the clock was ticking, I only had a couple of hours to work until it was time to switch back into mommy mode once the kids burst through the door. *Do I talk about the health benefits of self-pleasuring? Do I tell the story about how I bought my friends their first vibrators when we were seventeen? Or how my mom encouraged masturbation as a healthy and normal part of my teenage development?* Maybe . . . but then the writer's block settled in, and I sat there for a good twenty minutes while nothing came. So, I figured . . . *I would.*

This orgasm brought my entire body back to life, as I floated on a cloud of tingling, electric happiness. Anxiety immediately rushed out of my body as I was flooded with positive emotions. This simple act of self-pleasuring, or what I call a Solo Session, is my favorite means for shifting out of a lower, negative state and into a higher vibration (pun *definitely* intended) of loving consciousness and personal pleasure. I consider the Solo Session to be one of the greatest acts of self-love and self-care. Masturbating functions like a magic wand of sorts, a physical and emotional tool that opens up immediate creativity, flow, and magic in my life. With my regular self-pleasuring practice, my life-at-large is juicier, sweeter, more pleasurable, and more powerful. *This is the power of making love to yourself.*

I believe that how you feel about yourself sexually directly affects how you feel about yourself in every aspect of your life. If you're confident enough to touch yourself, you'll be more confident in your choices as a woman and as a mother. If you're free to express yourself during an orgasm, you'll feel freer to express yourself in a business meeting. If you feel empowered to give yourself pleasure, you'll feel empowered to ask for more pleasure in your relationship. In the words of Psalm Isadora, the departed tantra teacher and healer, *when you master your sexual energy, you gain mastery over your life.*

The Big O

There are a lot of reasons to give yourself more O's. Orgasms release your body's natural endorphins, ushering in a feeling of euphoria. They relieve stress by changing you from a negative to positive state in an instant—or however long it takes you to get there! Orgasms stir up stagnant energy in your body, releasing stuck emotions. A good, healthy orgasm connects you to yourself and gives your skin a natural glow. Masturbating can increase your sex drive by keeping you regularly revved up and in tune with your body. For mothers in particular, regular self-pleasuring is a practice in powerfully putting *your* needs first—even if just for a few moments.

As we dive deep into the experience of motherhood and take care of everyone else, it's easy to let time to ourselves fall by the wayside. And carving out space for self-pleasure? Forget it! Rarely does "Take five to masturbate" appear on your to-do list. Maybe you haven't touched yourself in years, maybe you ignore the desire when it arises. You've convinced yourself that you don't have the time. Worse, you're worried you'll get caught in the act by your kids, or that you need to save what little sexual energy you have for your partner. There's even a chance that guilt, shame, or embarrassment is lingering from your upbringing—maybe it was an act that was considered taboo, versus healthy and necessary.

Forget all that. You, Mama, have permission to self-pleasure. It's one of the most normal, healthy, honest, and healing acts of self-care you can do for yourself as a woman, mother, and partner. Generating your own sexual energy and power through self-stimulation is the rocket fuel, giving you the vitality and stamina you deserve. Plus, the better you understand your unique pathways to pleasure, the better you'll be able to communicate them to your partner.

The more O's you have, the easier and faster you will experience them, and the more you'll want to have them with yourself and your spouse. You're craving to rekindle a sensual connection to your partner ... it's part of what drove you to open this book. But before you can do that, you'll need to reignite and deepen that connection to yourself first.

Ask yourself: "How do I turn *myself back on?*" This is essential, though it's just the tip of the iceberg. Solo Sessions are an opportunity to explore answers to that question and more. All you have to do is make time.

. . . .

Solo Sessions make you happy.
They give you a minibreak from your responsibilities.
They remind you that you're a woman with desires.

. . . .

Welcome, Mama. This is your Solo Session, one of many Sexy Sessions you'll encounter throughout this book.

Sexy Session #1: The Solo Session

It's time to have a self-pleasuring Solo Session. You'll need five to fifteen minutes of privacy and perhaps, an awesome vibrator. Don't stress—there is absolutely no pressure on you, I promise. It may take thirty seconds to have an orgasm and you're done. Or, you might feel frustrated and find that you can't relax enough to even get there. You may take a deep dive into a fantasy and ride out twenty minutes of glorious pleasure. There's room for all of it! And then even more room to try again tomorrow, or the next day. It's all up to you, and it's all just for you.

I know you're a grown woman who's touched herself before, but just in case you need some inspiration for your Solo Session, here are a few tips:

1. Finding the Best Time for a Solo Session

You can squeeze in a self-pleasuring Session anytime you have a moment of privacy in your day. You don't *need* to schedule it, but you might want to if it will help you fit it into your busy routine. Here's a short list of opportunities to get down with yourself:

♥ Before your morning shower to start the day off right.

♥ Before you eat your lunch to work up an appetite.

♥ Before you take a nap to help you fall sleep.

♥ Before you do a home workout to get pumped up.

♥ Before you leave for school pickup to energize yourself for carpooling and activities with the kids.

♥ Before you leave for the grocery store so it doesn't feel like such a chore.

♥ When the kids are driving you crazy and you can escape from them for five minutes.

♥ In between conference calls, if you work from home, to take a short break and revive your energy.

♥ Immediately after you put the kids to bed to reset yourself for some grown-up time with your spouse.

♥ Basically anytime in the course of your day where you find yourself wasting your precious time and energy on social media.

2. Mojo Rising: Turning Yourself On

As you begin integrating the tools and exercises in this book, you'll start to see your sensual desire and "masturbation inspiration" naturally rise. However, the key to desire is not to wait for it to show up out of nowhere, but to *create it yourself*. For immediate desire-generating inspiration to get turned on for this Solo Session, you might:

♥ Massage your entire body with coconut oil, relishing in the smooth, slick texture as it glides over your skin.

♥ Dance slowly and seductively for yourself, caressing all your curves as you make your way to your bed.

♥ Read a sexy story, skipping straight to the good bits.

♥ Watch a seductive porn clip that presents women as equal sexual collaborators with men rather than as conquests. Do a quick Google search for "feminist porn" to begin your exploration. (See danabmyers.com/resources for more suggestions.)

♥ Press your favorite vibrator up against your body – outside of your clothes at first – and simply breathe into the sensations.

♥ Fantasize about the hottest sex you've ever had—with your husband or someone else.

♥ Watch as you touch yourself in the mirror.

3. Exploring Your Terrain

As you self-pleasure, pay attention to what feels good to you, because as they say, different strokes for different folks! As you try a few techniques, make mental notes of what's working for you, what's not, and what feelings are arising—good or bad. To begin, focus on arousing your whole body—bring in a silk scarf or feather to trace over your arms, belly, and thighs, slowly stimulating each part of your body as you prepare to journey toward orgasm. Or, give yourself a breast massage with coconut oil as a sensual warm-up. Here are ideas on how to touch yourself with pleasure:

♥ Making slow circles around your clitoris (or C-spot) with one finger, then adding in more fingers, one at a time, with varying pressure, until you're stroking with your entire hand. *Note: Your C-spot is the fleshy knob located just north of your vaginal opening. To find it, move toward the top of the labia but stay below your pubic bone. It's much like a penis in that during arousal it becomes engorged thanks to increased blood flow, and with this, becomes more and more sensitive to the touch.*

♥ Nestling your C-spot between two fingers, one on either side, stroking up and down, and side to side, exploring different intensities and rhythms.

♥ Tapping your vibrator or fingers lightly to your C-spot to build excitement, then exploring all of your labia and vagina before returning back up to your C-spot, creating a repetitive circular motion of total pleasure.

♥ Exploring your G-spot, a small spongy orb that's chock-full of nerve endings, located against the front wall of your vagina, about two inches inside the opening. To start stimulating, insert a finger (with your palm up toward your belly button) and make a come-hither motion with that finger against the front wall. There are also vibrators with curved arms specifically made to stroke the spot. Breathe deeply and see what sensations arise.

♥ Trying new positions on your back or belly, standing up or bent over the bed.

♥ Using your sex muscles and squeezing on your fingers or toy as you're building up your pleasure. Squeeze and release, then repeat, and explore how activating your Kegels (PC muscles) affects your journey to creating a stronger orgasm.

♥ Always remember to breathe and give yourself permission to vocalize the pleasure you're feeling: moaning, sighing, weeping, and howling are all natural and can help intensify your orgasmic release!

YOUR MISSION:
Commit to self-pleasuring once this week and every week that you continue to use the Mommy Mojo Makeover, in addition to the Sexy Sessions you'll be practicing with your partner. Believe in the power of pleasuring your pussy and make it a lifelong habit!

O-NOTES: KEEP A SEXY SESSIONS JOURNAL
Starting now, and continuing for the rest of this journey, you're going to journal about every Sexy Session. Include where and when you did it, what your inspiration was, what your orgasm felt like, and any other thoughts you have about the experience. You can elaborate or just keep it simple. It doesn't matter whether you make notes in your phone or a paper notebook, as long as you make them. Why? Because keeping notes will become a record of your progress and pleasure, and rereading those experiences is fun and encouraging. Anytime you're feeling *meh* about sex, you can look at your notes and be reminded of how great orgasms feel. Not sure how to get started? Here is an example from my own O-Notes to inspire you:

SATURDAY NIGHT

"We got home late from a party and C fell right to sleep. I still had energy and thought . . . why not have my own personal after-party? I laid down a towel in the bathroom in front of my full-length mirror and turned on my vibrating wand. I was on my knees, rising and falling and riding my toy, watching every move I made. It felt wild and even a little taboo with C sleeping in the next room. I squeezed my sex muscles and built up to a

truly electric, whole-body orgasm. In that moment, I wasn't a mother who had to get up in five hours with the kids. I was a rock star on stage, writhing with a 'microphone stand' between my legs until I shook and trembled with pleasure."

It's your turn, now! Write down a quick journal entry about your Solo Session:

_____

_____

_____

_____

_____

_____

_____

_____

_____

_____

_____

_____

_____

Reduce the Resentment

HE NEVER HELPS AROUND THE HOUSE.

He doesn't take the time to make me feel special anymore.

Why am I in charge of absolutely everything for the kids?

He goes to the gym after work, while I come home from work and go straight into doing dinnertime, homework, and bedtimes with the kids. It feels so unfair.

He never plans dates for us anymore, but then wants sex all the time. It's like he's forgotten I need some romance beforehand!

He thinks working full time is so much harder than what I do. It's infuriating that he sees my workload as a SAHM as somehow less than his. I want and need to feel more appreciated.

He leaves his laundry on the floor for me to pick up. It's as if he's another child I have to look after.

Do any of these gripes sound familiar? Were you nodding your head in agreement as you went down the list—with steam coming out of your ears?

The truth is that I've never met a mother who didn't harbor some kind of resentment toward her partner. Even though more fathers are sharing domestic and child-rearing responsibilities than ever before, it's hard to deny that women continue to take on more . . . and quite possibly, get thanked less. It's no surprise that resentment begins to fester. The internal fuming, the loop of muttered complaints that run through our minds on a daily basis—it's a terrible feeling, isn't it?

As Nelson Mandela said, "Resentment is like drinking poison and then hoping it will kill your enemies." But we all know it won't. Bottling up resentment in your relationship will only make YOU feel angry, sad, and disappointed. Worse, rekindling an intimate and enthusiastic sex life with your partner will feel almost impossible. Who wants to have sex when you're holding a grudge? You might even be thinking, "Why give him pleasure when he won't support me? I do everything around here!"

If left unaddressed, your resentment will simmer until it damages your friendship, strangles your sex life, and squeezes the life right out of your relationship. *Let's not let that happen, okay?*

There's still plenty of sex, love, and happiness to be had, so let's work on reducing resentment *today*.

ASK AND YOU SHALL RECEIVE

I know you want and deserve more help and recognition from your partner, so answer this question:

ARE YOU CLEARLY ASKING FOR WHAT YOU NEED IN A WAY THAT HE'LL RESPOND TO POSITIVELY?

Many of us don't ask in the first place—or we've stopped asking because we don't want to be perceived as a *nag*. On the flipside, some moms feel they *have* to do it all by themselves, as if that proves they're a good mother. Or, others just expect their spouses or partners to be mind readers.

Here's what I know: Your partner *wants* you to be happy. He wants you to feel energized and relaxed, sexy and supported. He doesn't want you feeling burdened with endless childcare, dishes, homework, and laundry. But people oftentimes need to be reminded to offer their support. They need to be given the opportunity to be your hero!

So how do you ask for what you need so that your man will hear you, respond positively, and give you the help you deserve?

The solution is so simple you won't even believe it:

WHEN ASKING FOR HELP, USE THE WORDS "WOULD" OR "WILL."

This simple-yet-ultra-effective communication tool is based on the advice of John Gray, Ph.D., relationship expert and author of *Men Are from Mars, Women Are from Venus*. Gray says that the most common mistake we make when asking for support is the use of the words "could" and "can" instead of "would" and "will." *Could you change the baby's diaper?* is an indirect question collecting information. Obviously, he *can*. He has two hands and knows how to fasten a diaper. *Would you please change the baby's diaper?* is a direct request that lets him know exactly how he can help you.

When you say "would you" or "will you," you're giving your spouse the opportunity to give you what you need, to be your hero in that moment. When you use the words "could you" or "can you," it comes across that they have no choice but to say yes, as though you're backing them into a corner with your demand. Gray also emphasizes the importance of being **brief and direct** in your requests, instead of lengthy and indirect, in order to make your message clear.

Trust me on this: using "would you" and "will you" is the first step to releasing the resentment you might harbor toward your spouse.

THE TOOL:
REDUCE THE RESENTMENT

Let's first look at a few examples of how to use this subtle shift in language to get your requests heard and delivered upon. Each example will give a "Do Say, Don't Say," and an explanation of why the shift in word choice makes such a profound impact.

Do Say: *Would you clear the disposal, babe?* (This is a clear, direct request that he can help you with.)
Don't Say: *The disposal is clogged. It's stinking up the whole kitchen. Can't you smell that?* (This is an irritated rant without a specific ask for help.)

Do Say: *Would you take me to a movie this week?* (This gives him a clear opportunity to fulfill your wishes.)
 Don't Say: *We haven't gone to a movie in weeks! Can you look online for what's showing?* (This carries a blaming tone, and fails to invite him to actually take you out.)

Do Say: *Will you tell me when you think I'm doing an amazing job at being a mom?*
(There's no shame in asking for recognition when you feel you're not getting it. He might just need a reminder!)
Don't Say: *You never tell me I'm doing a good job with the kids! Can't you just notice me?* (This is accusatory and doesn't offer a clear opportunity to fulfill your needs.)

Do Say: *Would you please do bedtimes tonight?* (This is brief and simple; and he doesn't actually need an explanation of why you want the night off.)
Don't Say: *I've done bedtimes for the last six days and I need to get to the gym because I feel fat and it's just your turn tonight!* (There's zero freedom of choice here!)

Do Say: *Babe, would you surprise me sometime with flowers or a love note? It would make me feel so loved and appreciated.* (This is an ultra-clear request for a romantic gesture that would make you feel good.)
Don't Say: *You never take the time to make me feel special anymore. Why can't you just bring me flowers or surprise me with a love note sometime?* (This is accusatory and doesn't set up him up in any way to be a loving hero!)

Do Say: *Will you put your laundry in the basket, babe?* (This is a direct request without any fluff or complaining.)
Don't Say: *Why is your laundry on the floor again? Don't you see the hamper sitting there?* (This is passive-aggressive and could escalate into a fight!)

I think you get the idea. It's a very subtle and simple thing, but it's really effective. Men respond to DIRECT REQUESTS—not demands or indirect requests.

Imagine it the other way around: If he said, *"Can you make dinner?"* Of course you can! You only do it every night! But if he said, *"Would you make me my favorite chicken dish tonight, babe?"* you'd feel completely different about it and see it as an opportunity to do something lovely for him, instead of seeing it as a chore.

. . . .

Mama's new magic words are
"would" and "will."
Use them to ask for what you want and need!

. . . .

YOUR MISSION:
USE "W-WORDS" TO REDUCE
YOUR RESENTMENT

Starting today, follow these six simple steps to more effectively ask for more support, recognition, and romance, and, therefore, start reducing the resentment that is sabotaging your relationship.

1. COMMIT TO ASKING AGAIN

Check in with yourself to see if you've been stuffing your resentment down, instead of giving him the opportunity to step up and help. If you notice that you've stopped asking for whatever reason, make the choice today to start asking for more support. Say it to yourself: *I will ask for more help in order to reduce my resentment.* Now, repeat it! Consider it your mission to invite him to be your helping hero, even if it's just the taking-out-the-garbage kind.

2. NOTICE IF YOU'RE USING C-WORDS

If you *have* been asking for help but are not getting it, take a moment to notice the language you've been using. If you find you're using "could" and "can," there's a good chance he hasn't exactly been racing to complete the task. What you want to ask is "will" he help support you. So, without any judgment, observe how often you use those C-words when you need something done. When I first did this exercise, I was *shocked* to see how often I threw down the C-words at my husband.

3. FIGURE OUT WHAT YOU WANT AND NEED

Next, figure out what kind of help will make you feel more supported, and how your spouse could make you feel more loved and appreciated. Do you need more help with childcare? Or for him to take on specific housekeeping duties without being reminded? To handle bedtimes twice a week so you can hit the gym or go on a girls' night? Do you want him to plan more date nights? Leave you love notes in your briefcase? Write your wants down in your journal, or say them out loud directly to your partner.

What do I want and need to feel supported by my partner?:

_____

_____

_____

_____

_____

_____

4. ASK FOR HELP USING W-WORDS

Pick *one thing* you need that would lessen your resentment toward him and make you feel more supported, appreciated, and loved— one thing that would make mom life feel easier and more joyful. **Then invite him to be your hero by asking for it using a brief, direct "would you" or "will you" question.** Remember, W-words present a clear request that someone can respond to. Refer to the examples above for inspiration, and for each request, write down what you would have said in the past, and what you will say now that you know the magic words. Writing these requests down, and even practicing them in the mirror, will reboot your confidence to ask for your needs to be met. Trust that your partner will rise up and deliver.

Do Say   **Don't Say**

_____   _____
_____   _____
_____   _____
_____   _____
_____   _____

5. EXPRESS YOUR GRATITUDE

When you ask for and get the support and appreciation you need, I beg of you: SHOW YOUR APPRECIATION! Express your gratitude loud and clear, in a heartfelt and generous manner. Even if *he* doesn't say thank you for all the little things you do; even if your inner bitch is silently screaming, *Shit, I don't get thanked every time I do a load of laundry . . . Why do I have to thank him?!* Calm that voice down. Isn't the end result of getting the help and recognition we crave worth thanking him for?

Let that resentment fall by the wayside and simply pour on loads of big, generous THANK YOUs when he says yes to your requests. More gratitude equals less internal fuming and creates space for more romantic feelings to bubble up . . . and that feels pretty amazing!

6. RESPECT HIS STYLE . . . AND RECIPROCATE!

If you ask him for help with the kids or with housekeeping, remember that he is not you. He can't do it like you—and you know what? He doesn't have to do it like you. Know that there will be backwards pajamas on the kids, unrinsed dishes in the dishwasher, or that compliment he gave you may not be a perfect line out of a romance novel. Breathe. It's okay that everything is not perfect. Cut him some slack and just relish the additional help and support you've asked for.

Now that you've learned to use the magic W-words and he's stepping up to the plate to be your hero . . . let's turn the tables and reciprocate. Consider how you may have contributed to the mutual resentment in your relationship. What does your partner resent you for? Can you encourage him to express it, so you can in turn change it and be a heroine for him? For true healing to begin, both parties need to take responsibility, communicate openly, and be willing to make changes in the dynamics of the relationship.

The Mommy Pop-Out

B EFORE I HAD KIDS, this is what freedom used to look like:

I spent countless hours walking around, taking in the sights and sounds of the city streets as the sun was setting. From Chicago to Los Angeles to Brooklyn, I wandered about after work with no specific destination in sight; popping in and out of shops, striking up conversation with strangers, marveling at public art, statues, and street performers.

I often received positive attention as I strutted down the block, and I always volleyed back a compliment in return. The whole experience was uplifting, flirtatious, and inspiring.

The mystery of what I might stumble upon next thrilled me endlessly. And like clockwork, exciting new ideas and connections formed, as sudden and striking realizations about life, love, and the future blossomed within me—all amidst that buzzing big city stimulation.

In my early life, this was my experience of being a woman in the world: free, fearless, flirtatious, playful, and curious. I was alone with my thoughts and I luxuriated in my unscheduled time—fully and completely. Until I had kids. And then, for a while, my great big world got a whole lot smaller; my time became strictly scheduled, my infinite possibilities suddenly seemed finite and limited.

Every mom out there knows that once we bear children, we relinquish ownership of our time. We are rarely free during those twilight hours between five and eight pm, as we are now chained to the homework + dinnertime + bath time + bedtime routine. This adorably-domestic-and-important-but-utterly-mundane daily pattern can leave us feeling drained, uninspired, and even captive to the responsibilities of family life.

Sure, bath time is sweet and story time is precious. However, being stuck inside the house every night, I started to feel like a caged animal: nothing new to see, all spontaneity lost to step-by-step routines. While having children had connected me to the world, it also isolated me from it. I felt like I was missing out on something. And then I realized I was missing the freedom, energy, and grown-up inspiration of those pre-kid walkabouts at dusk. It became clear to me that I had to get out, and it had to be during that window of time. I realized that my kids didn't really need me to do bath time every single night.

So I took back what was mine. I needed my autonomy to experience some unstructured time; to leave the house, to wander freely, and to explore the world once again. Plus, I needed a mental break from being *on* all the time! I needed the opportunity to exist only as *myself, as a woman*. And with the help of reliable childcare, I renamed my walks about town: The Mommy Pop-Out.

Once or twice a week, I started leaving the house for a mini two-hour excursion of uninterrupted me-time. I began "popping out" of the house from six-thirty to eight-thirty, to give myself a break from all that bath time and bedtime business. I wandered. I chatted. I even flirted a little. I browsed books and did hot yoga and had cocktails. I continually asked myself the questions, How sensually can I explore this moment? What are the sights, sounds, and smells right in front of me, ripe and ready to be devoured as inspiration? What does it feel like to claim these hours to "just be me," to engage my interests outside of motherhood and career? It was a luscious experiment in regenerating myself, in reclaiming my time and my personal freedom.

By the time I'd return home, the kids were already in bed. It was genius! I felt joyful, vibrant, rejuvenated, and sensual. I instantly became more passionate about myself, because let's face it, freedom is very, very sexy! As a bonus, I had more energy for sex on those nights, too. It was a revelation: a Mommy Miracle. I had effectively given myself permission to take the time I needed to be a real grown-up woman—and not just a parent. Even all these years later, not a week goes by where I don't take a Mommy Pop-Out. And now, it's your turn.

* * * * * * * * * * * * *

*Escape the mundane nighttime routine
and rediscover your sweet sovereignty with a Pop-Out!*

* * * * * * * * * * * * *

THE TOOL:
TAKE A POP-OUT, MAMA!

Once a week, starting now, you are going to take a Mommy Pop-Out: a two-hour escape into unadulterated me-time. That means you'll make a great escape from your domestic duties during the most hectic stretch of the day and dive into a short-but-sweet two-hour excursion to explore your world. You are going to lovingly pass the kids off to a sitter, your partner, a grandparent, or a friend you swap childcare with. And then, YOU GO OUT THE DOOR. Run, don't walk!

Here are some tried-and-true tips on how to actually make it happen:

1. ORGANIZE CHILDCARE A WEEK IN ADVANCE
In order to feel guilt-free about popping out, get your childcare plan in place first.

♥ Book a standing babysitter every week: same time, same place. Adjust your sitter's weekly hours to accommodate your excursion so you don't go over budget.

♥ Enlist your partner and give him a week's notice so he can prepare to be home at least fifteen minutes before you're set to leave. Once he sees how refreshed you feel upon returning home, he'll start volunteering to do the job every week.

♥ Prep the kids' dinner, homework, and jammies earlier in the day so there are no holdups to keep you from leaving.

♥ If you have no babysitting budget and your partner can't help, organize a childcare swap with a friend. She'll take your clan for your Pop-Out and you'll do her the same favor.

2. USE YOUR TIME WISELY (AND SENSUALLY!)
The beauty of the Pop-Out is that it's exclusively for inspiring and reviving yourself as a sensual woman. So, please don't spend your precious solo time picking up toilet paper at Target. Choose an excursion that stirs your sensuality, fills up your soul, and maybe even pushes

you out of your comfort zone. Engage in something that leaves room for curiosity, something that lights you up. Remember, you are capable of giving yourself the sensual energy you desire and deserve. Choosing an activity that sparks your sensual radiance is key to a successful Pop-Out. You might:

♥ Head to a bistro for an indulgent meal and journaling session. Flirting with the bartender is strongly encouraged!

♥ Wander aimlessly through that new neighborhood you're interested in—finally able to hear yourself think without being interrupted.

♥ Take a yoga class and stretch into the power of your own body, while your eyes feast on all those sexy sweaty bodies.

♥ Go to an author reading at the bookstore and ask a provocative question. Mingle with the other guests afterward and discuss.

♥ Take a pole dancing class (and wear the shoes!).

♥ Brainstorm that new business idea you've been thinking about for years, jotting notes on a napkin as you sip a martini.

♥ Meet a girlfriend for stiff drinks and get silly.

♥ Take a drawing, pottery, or painting class with your best friend, *avec wine*. Get your hands dirty and laugh until it hurts.

♥ Get your nails and toes done while reading an erotic novel (use your Kindle for privacy).

♥ Take a sketchpad or adult coloring book to a cozy cafe and rouse your inner artist.

3. POP BACK *IN*

The purpose of the Pop-Out is so you can pop back *in*—and reconnect to the sexy, interesting, smart, strong, and lit-up woman you truly are. When you take this time for yourself every week, you'll find that you return home feeling like the grooviest, most inspired, and empowered mother possible. And because you've freed yourself from one of the most exhausting routines of the day, you'll have more energy and enthusiasm to enjoy the rest of the evening with your partner, who you'll see as not just the person you parent with—but as your lover. You'll be so turned on by those two hours of freedom and inspiration that you just might have sex on the same night as your Mommy Pop-Out—and maybe it's *you* who initiates the action! It's a classic relationship win-win, but it's not just you and your partner who benefit. When you take time to yourself, you show your kids what it looks like to create healthy, self-nurturing habits. It's an important self-love tool that sets the example that you love yourself enough not to lose yourself. Truth: you're the *only one* who can give your children a happy mother who loves her life and owns her freedom. But you've got to do what you need to in order to make yourself happy.

NO EXCUSES: A note for moms who work full-time outside the house:

I understand that six-thirty to eight-thirty pm may be the only quality time you get to spend with your kids during the workweek. You may feel resistant to a Pop-Out—guilty even. But when you leave the office and head straight into SuperMom mode every single day, there's no time to decompress or connect with yourself. You may even find you're more short-tempered with the kids and your partner because of it. So, please, take a Pop-Out once a week. You deserve that breathing time! If it helps soothe the guilt, get home early enough to read the final bedtime story and you'll have the best of both worlds: quality inspiration time to yourself and bedtime snuggles, too.

BE HONEST . . . A note for moms who are already poppin' out:

If you already have plenty of me-time in your life, congratulations! But ask yourself this: Is your me-time *nurturing*? Do your Pop-Outs expand your *sensual* self and creativity? Can you try something slightly more exotic with your me-time, stretching beyond your current routine to discover something *new* about yourself? Take a look and see how you can up your Pop-Out game and make your me-time even more effective.

The Quickie
A Sexy Session

My husband: *Hi love. Meet me for a Quickie tonight?*

Me: *NOPE. I've been picking LICE out of our children's heads ALL after-noon. While you've been out enjoying YOUR life, I've been a NERVOUS WRECK. Actually, I think I hate you a little bit right now. I'm freaking out. Plus, I'm starving. I do NOT NEED A QUICKIE!*

My husband: *(silence)*

Me: *Hmm, maybe you're right... perhaps I DO need a Quickie.*

AND GUESS WHAT? I did. I really, *really* did. I put those lice-infested, shower-capped kids to bed and took a bath. I put my hands on my body and danced a little bit, readying myself for a hot Quickie that would literally flush the stress, agitation, and nervousness right out of me.

I gave and received a few moments of oral pleasure. I brought out the vibrator that gets me there in sixty seconds, *without fail*. It was amazing. It was *fun*. It took my mind off the "infestation" and the tension quickly melted from my body. I felt 100 percent closer to my husband than I did just an hour prior. I appreciated his effort to initiate the Sexy Session, making me feel desirable, even though I'd initially resisted the idea. The Quickie relieved my stress, gave me pleasure, and put me *back* on the same team as my husband. And all it took was ten minutes.

Sexy Session #2: The Quickie

Take charge of the pleasure and connection you crave by carving out time for a Quickie. This fast and intense Sexy Session is the perfect solution for parents short on time and sexual energy.

Let's face it: Quickies may have become your go-to source for sexual activity since you started having kids. But as the months and years have gone by, has the Quickie become the *only* sex you're having? That once-a-week, ten-minute, bare-minimum, routine romp you have every Saturday night just to hold your love life together? If that's the case, your once hot-and-heavy Quickie may have lost some of its initial luster, or worse, your sex life could be asleep at the wheel entirely.

With a hint of creativity and enthusiasm, and just a little bit of time, the Quickie can be an effective tool for awakening your sleepy sexual connection, and bringing back that electric, pre-parenting chemistry that once coursed through your veins.

• • • • • • • • • • • •

A Quickie is like an energy drink for your sex life,
but not your main meal.
There's just not enough sexual nutrition to sustain and nourish you both!

• • • • • • • • • • • •

YOUR MISSION: HAVE A QUICKIE

Your mission is to have an intense, fast frolic with your spouse or partner. Together, you'll focus on generating more passion and excitement than any sex you've had in the past few months. No longer will your Quickie be the lackluster "mandatory sex" you have every Saturday night. This Session is designed to infuse a more potent and powerful sexual energy into your routine sex life.

Below are some guidelines to make this Quickie much hotter than usual:

1. TO PLAN OR NOT TO PLAN?

Unlike other Sexy Sessions you'll read about later, the Quickie doesn't require any elaborate planning. You can grab your partner for this Session whenever you see a window of opportunity. For example, right before the kids wake up or after they've fallen asleep, or even sneaking away while they're occupied with their homework. But let's be honest, Mama: How many times have you *seen and seized that kind of opportunity* lately? Answer: Probably not too often. While spontaneously initiating a lustful Quickie may be the ultimate goal, most mamas prefer a hint of planning so that both parties are ready and willing to get down to business.

Pick a time when you'll be able to be present without distractions, and then communicate that to your partner. Yes, that could mean you'll have to muster the energy after the kids are asleep, but since you'll know this in advance, you'll be able to mentally prepare for it. Take a nap, have an extra cup of coffee, or squeeze in an energizing workout to fuel your body and mind with sustaining energy (remember, you only need ten minutes for this—you *can* find the time). Try a bit of virtual foreplay to build anticipation a few hours prior. Engage in sexy texting banter to let each other know what you have in mind for later. Your first text might read something like, *"Excited to see you in the bedroom at ten sharp for ten minutes of pleasure. I'll be naked."*

2. HEAT THINGS UP QUICKLY

With a Quickie, there's less time to get turned on. To heat up the action and get your mind and body in the game fast, run through this checklist:

- ♥ Remove any children's toys from your location. Stepping on Legos and staring at stuffed animals is a sexual no-no.
- ♥ Play a fantasy out in your mind, or read a few pages of an erotic book, before you get started. When your mind is aroused, your body should follow.
- ♥ Touch yourself for five to ten minutes beforehand to boost your arousal. If possible, bring yourself to the brink of an orgasm, but hold back. You'll be that much closer to the Big O when your Quickie begins.
- ♥ Have your favorite lubricant and vibrators close at hand and use them right away.
- ♥ Put on a playlist with a sexy edge or a driving beat.
- ♥ Place your partner's hands exactly where you want them and be honest about what *really* does it for you. If being on top or taken from behind will bring you to orgasm faster, tell him. Encourage him to do the same.

3. INFUSE FIERY PASSION

To banish the boredom and breathe sexy, stimulating new life into your Quickie, consider these few tips:

♥ Leave on your work skirt or nightie, with no undies underneath. There's something seriously sexy about leaving on a few bits of clothing during a fast and furious romp.

♥ Introduce a new couples' toy, like a vibrating C-ring, into the Session. The novelty will feel exciting to you both and the buzz can help you reach orgasm faster.

♥ Slip into a pair of heels and crotchless panties or other lingerie accessories that you both find libidinous.

♥ Choose a new location to get busy: on top of the washer, in the garage or home office or the garden, patio, or shower. A simple change in environment can heighten eroticism.

♥ Take control. If you're usually more demure during sex, assume a bolder, more assertive moxie. You choose the position and move him there *with your body*. Then, switch it up again.

♥ Add in a new prop for sensory stimulation. Think blindfold or scarf to cover the eyes, or a tickler or spanker to excite the skin.

♥ Take turns giving and receiving oral pleasure or manual pleasure. Let it be fast, furious, hungry, and enthusiastic. Quickies *are* quick, but they aren't just about intercourse!

♥ Stand in front of a mirror and watch yourselves be carnal. It's nothing short of *hot*.

♥ Be more vocal. Moaning with pleasure when something feels good can build momentum. If the kids are in the house and you're concerned they'll hear you, turn on some music to drown out the sound, or simply murmur quietly into your partner's ear.

♥ Do it when there's a chance you'll get interrupted (but lock your door so the kids don't catch an eyeful!) This can up the excitement and bring back a hint of dangerous energy.

TO COME OR NOT TO COME

Because this is a Quickie, there's no anxiety that needs to be had. He's not worrying about how long he has to keep going, and you can be present without thinking about what's next on your to-do list. The same goes for reaching orgasm. Whether it's oral pleasure, or using your vibrator in advance, do what stimulates and excites you quickly. But, don't get hung up on reaching the Big O. Focus on experiencing pleasure and the feeling of your bodies colliding together in a more animalistic expression instead. If an orgasm comes, it comes; take the pressure off the outcome and enjoy the moment.

Does this sound good?

It's possible you're either nodding along in agreement, or you're shaking your head thinking . . .

What is this lady talking about? How am I supposed to conjure an instantaneously passionate, wild-and-wanton energy when I hardly have ANY sex drive AT ALL?

I hear you, and I understand. A wanton Quickie might sound a little crazy just a few days into this journey together. But the secret is this:

YOU FAKE IT 'TIL YOU MAKE IT

No, you don't need to fake an orgasm, or *force yourself* to do anything that feels uncomfortable. However, if you suspend any current beliefs that you are sexually uninspired and lack desire, then you'll have the mental capacity for a can-do attitude. For the moment, just act out of character and engage in joyful pretend play. Decide to embody the turned-on vixen instead of the tired-out mom.

Here's some inspiration for how to do just that:

♥ Conjure up the hottest sex you ever had with your partner (which was probably when you first met) and try to physically and emotionally recall why that felt *so* good.
♥ If that doesn't do it for you, try remembering the hottest sex you ever had with someone else. Remember how you felt in that moment, how every cell was at attention, awaiting the next kiss, touch, and thrust.
♥ Or, take your imagination further and picture yourself as an exotic, highly sought after queen or bad-ass superheroine—or any kind of fantasy figure or archetype that invokes a feeling of bona fide, empowered sensuality. Channel *that* energy, and imagine that this sex appeal already exists inside of you.

As parents in a long-term relationship, it's rare to find yourselves so authentically turned on that you just have to jump each other's bones for a filthy, passionate Quickie. But, remember . . . YOU CAN CREATE THAT. All you have to do is start bringing it to the table, even if it feels as though you're playing at first.

Believe that you're making love like it's the last time you'll ever get to. Kiss your partner like there's no tomorrow! Yes, it may feel awkward at first, but before you know it, that "acting" will soon turn into your reality. Once you're reminded of how good it feels to be *that* passionate, you'll start believing that you really can become that steamy and spontaneous once again. So, go on and use this kind of "passionate play-acting" to reawaken the liveliness and vivacity that your early relationship Quickies once had.

O-NOTES: A SEXY SESSIONS JOURNAL

It's time for more O-Notes! Once you've had your Quickie, jot down where and when you did it, who initiated, what your inspiration was, what your orgasm felt like (if you had one), and any other thoughts you had about the experience.

Write down a quick journal entry about your Quickie:

_____

_____

_____

_____

_____

_____

_____

_____

_____

_____

_____

_____

_____

_____

_____

_____

_____

Choose Fun over Obligation

WHEN WAS THE LAST time you used the word "fun" to describe your daily life as a mom?

Is it fun to clean up toys, be thrown up on, prepare meals and snacks, potty train, teach manners, run errands, carpool, help with homework, wrangle wild things into bed, and monitor a teenager's social media account . . . all while juggling a career and your relationship? The short answer: Not so much.

This letter submitted to my website, from Abby, a mom of one, illuminates this issue perfectly:

Dear Dana,

Having a loving husband, my own business, and a baby girl is truly my dream come true, but if I'm honest, it doesn't always feel so dreamy. My girl is three, and I thought I'd be so much more in-the-moment with her. Instead, it feels like I'm roboti-

cally "plugging in the pieces" of our day. I'm always looking ahead to what's next—a meal, activity, bath, bedtime, etc.—so much so that I miss out on the sweetness of "what's happening now." I see other moms having FUN with their kids and it makes me sad. I'm even ashamed to admit that I often feel angry about it. I was also raised to believe that you have to finish your work before you play. And my work—both as her mom and as an entrepreneur growing my business—is never done, so I never allow myself to fully get to the "play part" of motherhood. This leaves me feeling stuck in stress mode and isolation, and it's certainly not making magic happen in my relationship with my husband either.

Please, please tell me . . . how can I enjoy motherhood more? I desperately want to be a happier mama, woman, and wife!

XO, Abby

I could totally relate to Abby's predicament. I often struggled to experience the joy "in the moment" with my kids—my mind would inevitably drift to work deadlines or other domestic obligations. While I hate to admit it, I often found the minutiae of motherhood *boring*, which only made me feel guilty. On top of that, I was mentally and emotionally exhausted from constantly shifting between the roles of mother and businesswoman. For me, trying to be everything to everyone at every single moment, meant that I missed out on the joy of being in the here and now. What's worse is that this inner discord also affected my marriage and sex life. I was often restless, resentful, and unhappy at the end of the day, and my husband was getting the bare minimum from me—whatever was leftover. Don't get me wrong, I've always loved being a mother, but there were times I was downright irritated and overwhelmed by the endless obligations that came with it. Let me tell you something: obligation is So. Not. Sexy.

I wanted to unearth bliss within the chaos, rediscover delight in the precious moments with my children, and find a way to make my life a whole lot of *fun* again! Something had to shift and I had a hunch it would have to be my attitude. That's when it came to me in a flash, like a light bulb going off in my brain:

- ♥ I decided I would CHOOSE FUN, whenever possible.
- ♥ I would choose PLEASURE over a sense of obligation.
- ♥ I would choose SILLINESS over boredom.
- ♥ I would choose AMUSEMENT over irritation.
- ♥ I would choose MY MOM TRIBE over isolation.
- ♥ I would choose to SEEK SENSUALITY over strict scheduling.

This radical change in mind-set was a revelation. I realized that, amidst all the chaos and sleeplessness, there is magnificence to be had in motherhood. Why miss out on it? Why not squeeze the pleasure and bliss out of every single moment?

Even with this new attitude, I still had to run the household and get my work done, change stinky diapers and operate on less than six hours of sleep, but I decided I would do it with more merriment. I'd listen to more music, find the humor in the madness of it all, and eat more chocolate along the way. I'd abandon my strict by-the-minute schedule and opt for a more spontaneous family flow. I'd attend more playdates with friends, even if it meant I had to leave work early and finish up once the kids were in bed. Fun would be *my choice*. And it worked! Motherhood became much more fun. I became much more like my old self again. The moments spent doing the simplest of things with my kids became so much sweeter, so much more amusing. I began to get my glow back, and feel like me again. I freed myself of the unnecessary feelings of anger and obligation that were plaguing me, and my Mojo began to steadily rise. Motherhood became more joyful, and that newfound happiness carried right over into my relationship.

I shared this personal success story with Abby and, inspired by my process, she began to focus her attention on finding more fun and pleasure, and her experience of motherhood changed for the better.

. . . .

Fun is the gateway drug to happiness.

. . . .

Mama, pleasure and fun are your birthright—they are yours for the taking. That's not to say that holding onto this lighthearted mind-set is always easy, but it is worth it. When you're having more fun within the daily grind of motherhood, your whole life will become happier. Fun offsets exhaustion; fun is a way out of feeling blue. Fun melts away fear, doubt, and stress. Fun can keep you from unleashing your inner tyrant upon your kids and husband. Fun makes room for present moment magic with your kids, opening your eyes to the possibility of more pleasure in *all* areas of your life—including in the bedroom! Choose fun every day, and you will access your glow once again.

Since there is never a better time than *now* to enjoy motherhood, here are some ways you can start practicing how to choose fun every single day:

1. Tap into the Power of PMA

PMA is your Positive Mental Attitude. Your thoughts are the most powerful tools you've got, and it's important to remember that you are *always* in control of them. Your thoughts shape your reality. If I was ever negative about something as a child, my mother would always chuckle and say, "Use your PMA, baby!" While I'm sure I did some serious eye-rolling at the time, her coaxing always helped me shift my thinking toward a more optimistic approach to the situation at hand.

We all tell ourselves a certain story, and our stories as we perceive them become our truths. So, if the stories of your life as a mom often start with a begrudging "I have to," it's time to let that go and write a new story. Instead of viewing the tasks of motherhood as obligations, how can you see them as opportunities for fun? Here's something to try: replace "I have to" with "I get to."

Here are some examples of replacing your obligated "I have to's" with pleasure-filled "I get to's":

♥ ***I have to*** *cook a week's worth of meals this morning.*
♥ ***I get to*** *listen to favorite music and savor the fresh scents of the food I'm making.*

♥ ***I have to*** *pack so much crap and then drag it all the way to the play-ground.*
♥ ***I get to*** *watch them play and laugh in the sandbox, and maybe even read a few pages of my book with an iced coffee in hand.*

♥ ***I have to*** *spend my whole afternoon at soccer practice.*
♥ ***I get to*** *hang on the sidelines with my girlfriends and catch up on each other's lives.*

♥ *I have to* listen to them scream my name a thousand times when I really need to finish up these work emails!

♥ *I get to* hear them call ME "mommy." This is a greater gift than finishing my emails can give me!

When you change how you see *and* say things, it changes the dynamics and instantly gives you a boost of positivity. Consistently using this tool will encourage you to become more present and enjoy even the most mundane moments of motherhood. Although it's a very simple shift,

---

Note: I'm not suggesting you *fake* happiness when you're feeling lonely and bored to tears, or missing out on a play date because you're holed up at the office racing to meet a deadline. It's not mandatory to enjoy motherhood all the time. And certainly, *faking it* is no good. I'm just trying to help you organically *find* more happiness within many of the moments you have no control over, because the moment is all you have.

---

it'll dramatically reduce the frustration and resentment you may be harboring. You'll be happier—and happiness feels pretty damn sexy.

Now, it's your turn. Take a moment to write down your most frequent "I have to" statements, and then transform them into "I get to's."

I HAVE TO . . .	I GET TO . . .

2. Ditch Obligations and Choose Fun Instead

As a mom, there are things we are *obligated to* do—and then, there are things we can choose to ditch. I want you to look for opportunities to ditch something that doesn't contribute to your happiness, and use that time to create more opportunities for fun instead.

For example, if you can't stand Sports Day at school, and your kids aren't passionate about it either, then do everyone a favor and just skip it. Take them out of school for the day and go on an adventure to a museum, a historical tour of the city, or even to the beach instead. Wear matching hats and be as silly as you can be together, skipping down the street or rolling down the grassy hill in the park. Feeling exasperated with all the laundry that needs to be folded? Leave it to sit for another day, and whisk everyone off for a movie and popcorn. Don't feel like pulling yourself off the couch to bathe them? Skip it (if they're not filthy, of course!) and play a game of Connect Four with them while you nurse a cocktail. If mommy-and-me classes bore you to tears, go out for a weekday champagne brunch with your baby in the stroller. I promise you, there is *always* a mom friend up for this one. Like you, she's just waiting to give herself permission!

It's not just boring kid stuff you have permission to ditch either. Hate ironing? If you can, tweak your budget and gleefully send your dress shirts down the street to the dry cleaners. Can't bear wasting a whole day inside waiting for the dishwasher technician to come? Leave it for another day and go break a well-deserved sweat at the gym. Sick and tired of eating so healthy? Go out and get the biggest burger you can find—a little indulgence every now and then is good for you! Finished your work, but feel guilty leaving the office early? Drop it, and spend the afternoon reading trash magazines at a local cafe.

You *always* have a choice, so why not choose to be amused and exhilarated in some way, each and every day? Knowing you always have that choice is empowering, and owning that choice feels incred-ibly sexy.

What does choosing more fun look like to you? Give yourself "Permis-sion to Ditch" and jot down specific ways you could ditch the dull and choose fun instead:

_____

_____

_____

_____

Choosing Fun Every Day

With the power of PMA and permission to ditch now firmly placed in your tool kit, take one final moment to consider how you can bring more fun, silliness, laughter, and sensual pleasures into your daily expe-rience. Maybe you slowly savor a delicious bite of sea-salted dark choco-late the next time you read them that story they love for the hundredth time. Maybe you take an evening family walk under the stars, catching lightning bugs in glass jars. Or pump up the volume and dance wildly while you assembly-line the dishes after dinner. Wear bright red lipstick to school pickup and dish out compliments to the other moms you see. And, of course, you can do the obvious and blast "Girls Just Want to Have Fun" in your car while you carpool.

You're a mom now, so embrace the fact that you might be a hot mess for a while, and since that's the case, you may as well try and have as much fun as possible while you're in the thick of it. There is pure, present moment joy accessible to all of us. Saying YES to having more fun within the mundane will transform your life. You just have to make the choice!

Take Time to Meditate

*C*HOCOLATE. WINE. MY VIBRATOR.

These are just a few of the trusty tools I rely on to help me navigate the chaotic, multitasking marathon of motherhood. But often I need to go deeper to disconnect from mommy madness and reconnect with my Mommy Mojo. That's when I turn to Sexy Mama Meditation and Mojo Mantras.

Before I became a mom, I used meditation to handle the stress of running a business and to cultivate confidence before speaking engagements. When I became pregnant, I meditated to connect to my physical wisdom and power in preparation for a natural birth with my son. With my second pregnancy, when my daughter turned breech at thirty-two weeks, I meditated to soothe some pretty intense fears surrounding the planned C-section. No matter the circumstance, the practice has always encouraged me to find more peace, happiness, and clarity in each moment, and certainly, to judge myself less and love myself more. Whether it's been learning in-person meditations at yoga class or listening to guided meditations online, the experience has been nothing short of transformative.

But since having kids, I've discovered that the big bonus of a meditation practice—albeit, one with a slightly sexy spin—is that it has dramatically helped boost my sexual desire and inspired better sex with my hubby.

Yes, you read that right.

I believe that great sex requires us to quiet our racing minds and become more present in our bodies. Being present helps us to relax and become more receptive and responsive to pleasure. Those long, slow breaths you practice in meditation are the same long, slow breaths you can use during lovemaking to help you become more aware of the sweet sensations that are arising. Meditation is simply good practice for being more present and mindful in your sex life.

The opposite holds true as well. If you kick off a Sexy Session and your mind is running over a twelve-point list of all the things you need to do, you've removed your *presence* and taken yourself *out* of the moment. You've allowed distraction to disconnect you from your partner and robbed yourself of your own pleasure, too.

Turn on Your Brain, Turn on Your Body

As a new mom, your whole world is turned joyously upside down, and there are simply more important things to think about than sex (like, keeping another human alive!). You think, *this will pass, I'll get a handle on it, and my sex life will naturally bounce back*. But as the kids get older, they need you even more. There isn't some miracle moment by which there is suddenly an abundance of time and space to put loads of thought into renewing your sex life. The truth is that if you stop thinking about your sensuality and sex life, it dries up. It falls off your radar and out of your relationship—and quick. To put amazing sex back into your relationship, you've got to put it back on your brain.

But, as a busy and often distracted mama, we need a *practice* that wakes our minds up out of its sexual lethargy. We need a few tools that get sex and sexiness back on our brains.

Think about it: the reason your children are so awesome is because you're thinking about them all the time. All that thought leads to positive action that nurtures and grows bright, compassionate, talented, beautiful little humans. So, imagine how awesome and vibrant your sexual energy could become if you gave it just a fraction of the mental energy you put toward your kids!

We'll kickstart these thoughts with a Sexy Mama Meditation called Sensual Daydreaming. This tool is used to reduce stress, increase relaxation, upgrade your inner hotness, and become more alive in your sexual energy. It's part meditating, part fantasizing, and definitely a little spicier than your average relaxing meditation. It gets your Mojo moving in the right direction, and all it takes is ten minutes.

A SEXY MAMA MEDITATION: SENSUAL DAYDREAMING

Think of this meditation as a trip down memory lane—the sexiest, most satisfying memory lane you can dream up. The perfect time to dive into this meditation is several hours before you initiate a Quickie, or on a morning where you foresee an opportunity for a Solo Session before school pickup. Meditating hours before any kind of Sexy Session *is* the secret! When you set a steamy intention with this sexy meditation long before it's time to get naked, you create space for sensual thoughts to dance and play . . . *all day long*. Naturally your body will begin to respond to those thoughts—with excitement, anticipation, and a steadily rising libido. You'll find you're so much more aroused, awakened, and enthusiastic for your Sexy Sessions when the seduction begins. Think of it like private mental foreplay *before* your foreplay!

These next ten minutes are for you alone, so drop in deeply and enjoy every moment. All you need is *you*. A note: read through the entire meditation completely before trying it out on your own. Don't stress out about remembering it all—you can keep opening your eyes to read each step, and then close your eyes again. Eventually, you'll get the hang of it and won't need to refer to the next set of instructions at all.

To begin, sit or lie down on a yoga mat or your bed—wherever you can feel the most comfortable and relaxed. If you'd like, turn on a playlist full of seductive songs to set the mood.

♥ Close your eyes and take a deep, glorious breath in. Exhale with a fantastic sigh.

♥ Slowly, deeply, breathe in again, a bit deeper this time. Your belly expands out, your lungs open wider. Exhale with a great, cleansing sigh.

♥ Let go of any thoughts, your to-do list, any stresses of the moment, the day, the week. Let go fully as you exhale again, with a melting sigh.

♥ Inhale and expand your beautiful belly. Breath rises up to fill your lungs wider, more open. Pause here at the top and exhale with a gentle sigh.

♥ Place your right hand on your lower belly, the place of your sexual energy. As you make contact, see a deep orange glowing ball of light below your palm, growing stronger and brighter. Inhale and exhale as it grows rich and vibrant in your belly, and then slowly spreads deep into your hips and all the way down to your feet. Continue inhaling and exhaling.

♥ Place your left hand over the center of your heart, the place of unconditional love. Visualize a sparkling, electric emerald green light radiating in your chest, spreading like wild moss through your shoulders and arms, out through your fingertips. Continue inhaling and exhaling.

♥ Become aware of your skin. With your fingertips, slowly touch the skin of your arm. First, the outside. Then, turn your arm over and run your fingers along the inside. You are soft, supple. You are responsive. Feel a sensual energy begin to rise in your body again and move through you. Just be curious. Continue inhaling and exhaling.

♥ Lift your fingertips to your neck. Feel your skin as if your fingertips belonged to your lover. Explore. One fingertip, two, three. Touch the side of your face, behind your ear, the small of your neck. Continue inhaling and exhaling.

♥ Bring your fingertips to your breasts. Feel your the weight of them in your hands, the pulse of your femininity in your heartbeat. Give them a tender caress, tracing pleasurable circles around your nipples. Continue inhaling and exhaling.

♥ Glide your hands down to where your thighs meet your Sex. Then, bring one hand to cup your Sex, and place your other hand on top. Offer your pussy a little hit of pleasure by adding some gentle pressure. Continue inhaling and exhaling.

♥ Now, you are awake. You are wanting. Something beautiful has begun to awaken inside you and your blood begins to move. Your energy is moving, rising through your body. Continue inhaling and exhaling.

♥ Now, conjure the memory of the hottest, most satisfying, most pleasurable, most gratifying, soul-shaking, life-changing sexual experience you ever had, with your spouse or a former lover. There should be no guilt or shame in your heart when thinking about a former lover, it's merely a healthy fantasy—a seductive, mental daydream, *not* a betrayal. So, don't censor the visuals that come to you. *Allow them to flow.* Maybe it is the sex you had in the sea on vacation, or it might be a raw, intense moment you had in a freight elevator. Keep inhaling and exhaling.

♥ Replay it all in your mind. Where were you? Was it dark or light outside? Was it raining? What did your lover do that turned you on so much? What did the sex smell like, feel like, taste like? How did it begin . . . and how did it end? Go deep into the visualization and see if you can *feel* absolutely everything that what was happening then, in that moment, in your body *now*. Breathe into this powerful memory, into the physical, emotional, and even spiritual connection you felt at that moment.

♥ Continue to recall this experience as completely as you can. Every nuance. How does your body feel right now? Do you feel arousal? Is your heart beating faster? Put your hands on your body again if you feel called to. Breathe in and out, allowing the memory to wash through you.

♥ Breathe in again, deeply. Bring your arms out to your sides, opening your palms to the sky. Expand your belly. Exhale, release.

♥ It is time to return to the room you are in, just as you are. Rub your palms together briskly, place them softly over your closed eyes, and very slowly lift them away. Gradually open your eyes as you lift your hands away, slowly bringing light back into your sight.

Welcome back, Mama. How was that? Can you feel the stirring sensual power behind this meditation? The magic it worked to relax your body and mind, while stimulating authentic arousal?

YOUR MISSION:

Try this practice out once or twice a week, on a day you've scheduled a Sexy Session, or when you wake up with a little tingle down below. Experiment with different "flavors" of this daydream: imagine a scenario with your spouse, partner, a past "bad boy" lover, a celebrity crush, or the hot single dad you spotted at the park. Anyone can be fodder for this sexy meditation!

If you feel moved, flow right into a Solo Session. Or hold off and allow the arousal and anticipation to grow throughout the day until your partner comes home. Sensual Daydreaming creates a space for exciting and lustful thoughts to play, and when you practice this Mojo Meditation, you'll see that your entire world starts to feel sexier and more pleasurable.

MOMMY MOJO MANTRAS

Now, I know that you may not always be able to stop, drop, and do a Sexy Mama Meditation—you may have babies hanging on your every limb or are running from meeting to meeting at work. But you can always give your Mojo a mini-shot of meditative inspiration and sensual self-empowerment with an on-the-go Mommy Mojo Mantra. A mantra is a word or series of words repeated to aid concentration in meditation, and can either be said out loud or silently. You can use a Mojo Mantra at any moment: right before a Sexy Session, in the throes of a body confidence crisis, when you feel like you're failing as a mom, or even, right smack in the middle of sex.

I have one Mojo Mantra that has stuck with me for a few years, and it works in just about every situation. It's a little bit magic in that way. Here's the story of how it came to be:

It was the night of my first live Mommy Mojo Makeover workshop in Brooklyn. I'd sold tickets, packed goodie bags, rehearsed the exercises, and had a hot, underwear-clad, male model waiting in the wings to read the moms some steamy erotica. I was excited! But as I set up the venue, my excitement turned into gut-wrenching nervousness. *Who was I to teach this workshop, when I myself was still figuring out how to reignite my own sex life after two babies? Why did I stuff myself into these jeans? Wait, are the kids going to love the nanny more than me?* I began to feel nauseous and totally doubt myself. In that moment, I knew I had a choice: pack up and go home, or pull myself together and deliver an amazing moms' night out for the women who had purchased tickets. In that instant, I began to chant a new mantra:

. . . .

I am calm, I am capable, I am confident.

. . . .

Then, for good measure and added sex appeal, I looked in the mirror and added:

And I'm fucking hot!

Over and over, I began repeating it, at first silently and then out loud.

I said it over and over until the panic subsided and I felt *calm, capable, confident, and HOT.*

My Mommy Mojo Mantra worked like a charm. The night was a success. The mantra gave me the power I needed in that moment and a renewed sense of belief in myself. I became empowered to inspire others to feel the same way.

THE TOOL:
CREATE YOUR OWN MOMMY MOJO MANTRA

Now, it's time for you to write your own personal Mommy Mojo Mantra: a unique phrase that addresses what you need to reconnect with yourself, ignite your sensuality, and bring you into the present moment.

Here are a few examples to get your creativity flowing:

When you need to let go of distraction and be present during sex . . .

♥ **I deserve pleasure. I crave this connection. I welcome this moment with my lover.**

When you can't zip up your pants and are feeling unsexy . . .

♥ **I am beautiful, sensual, and unselfconscious, right here, right now, in this body.**

When you're feeling "less than" or comparing yourself to others . . .

♥ **I am desirable and powerful simply for being myself!**

When you're feeling like your professional or creative dreams got pushed aside by motherhood . . .

♥ **I am just getting started. I have plenty of time to pursue my dreams!**

When you feel as though your sex drive will never, ever return . . .

♥ **I am a sexual being and have what it takes to give and receive pleasure. My sex life is a work in progress!**

When you're feeling guilty for taking me-time . . .

♥ **I can't take care of my children unless I take care of myself.**

When you're so exhausted that you lose your temper in front of your kids . . .

♥ **I'm human and I forgive myself. It was a bad moment, but I'm not a bad mother.**

When you feel resentful toward your partner because you're taking on too much domestic work . . .

♥ **When I ask for help, I will get the help I need.**

YOUR MISSION: CREATE YOUR OWN MOMMY MOJO MANTRAS

Take a few moments to brainstorm some Mojo Mantras. First, identify the frequent Mojo Blocks you experience that invoke your inner critic (when I feel X), and then write out a few mantras in response to counter the negativity, discomfort, distraction, etc. Keep your list going until you unearth the mantras that calm your nerves, boost your sexy self-confidence, and really get your Mojo rising.

When I feel: _____

Mojo Mantra: _____

When I feel: _____

Mojo Mantra: _____

When I feel: _____

Mojo Mantra: _____

When I feel: _____

Mojo Mantra: _____

Now, share it with a member of your Mom Tribe!

Once you've got your new mantras locked down, call another mom and tell her about it. Sharing is an amazing way to reinforce what you've learned and to inspire other moms in your life to do the same. You can even guide her through the process to create her own.

· · · · · · · · · · · · ·

Mama, you're now well on your way to becoming a more satisfied and stimulated mother and partner. In part two, prepare to arouse your sensual energy through movement, rally your Mom Tribe for a playful excursion, and voice your deepest desires in a loving conversation with your partner. You'll even continue to stoke the fires of passion with your lover with two more empowering Sexy Sessions. Prepare to up the game!

· · · · · · · · · · · · ·

PART TWO

• • • • • • • • •

Shake Up Your Mojo

• • • • • • • • •

Dance to Ignite Your Sensuality

"**M**OTHERHOOD IS GREAT FOR** your libido!" *said no one, ever.*

Let's face it: Moms are overtired, overcommitted, and overstimulated. The intensity of the day-to-day grind of motherhood can suck the sensuality right out of you, sapping your inner radiance and flatlining your libido. And, if you're like most moms, you may also feel a little depressed about your body after birth.

But there's a very simple tool that's *always* available for you to shake off the stress, infuse your soul with radical energy, and confidently reconnect you to yourself. You'll be up close and personal with your body in a way you haven't been since the kids came along, and that's a total turn-on.

It's DANCE, and it's the perfect antidote to balance the highs and lows of being a mom while unapologetically accepting and embracing your body as the sexiest on the planet.

Let's take Elissa's story, for instance, a stressed-out, under-sexed mom. In her own words, Elissa illuminates the transformative power that dance had on her journey toward getting her Mommy Mojo back:

"Anxiety is something I've experienced throughout my life and it's intensified since having my two babies. I'm overwhelmed with a thousand worries daily about being a mom. Am I giving the kids the best food? Should they be reading by now? Am I spending enough time with them? What if they're bullied? And then, the thought about my own body begin: Why can't I control what I eat? How am I still 10 pounds up? The racing thoughts got so bad on one morning - I woke up in a panic, my breath constricted and my body seized up with tension. I took ten deep breaths, I journaled, I hugged my husband. And then, I knew what I needed to do. I brought myself to a dance class at S-Factor, the pole studio I attend. And I had the most transformative, powerful, sensual dance session ever! I walked into the studio as one woman— anxious, nervous, fearful, shaky—and I walked out another. I felt free. Calm. Sweaty. Alive. Powerful. Grateful for the love in my life. Grounded and sexy in my perfectly imperfect body. What came to me through dancing is not to hate my anxiety and wish it away . . . but to embrace it, to love it, to physically move into it. Because by moving into it through dance, I was able to move out of it."

Oh, yes, mama. This is the power of dance, and it's a tool you can use every single day to soothe, empower, express, ignite, and even forgive yourself. Here's how you can put some dance into your day:

♥ In the morning as you transition from frantic-mom-trying-to-get-her-kids-to-school mode into hot-boss-mom-ready-to-take-on-the-day mode.

♥ Before a moms' night out, to get amped up for cocktails, chatter, and flirtation with your mom tribe.

♥ Before a difficult conversation with your partner, or after you've had an argument. It helps to release tension and create space within for honest communication and connection.

♥ While watching TV before bed, to sensually stretch out sore muscles from carrying groceries and backpacks and kids all day.

♥ After you've lost your temper with the kids, dance as an embodiment of prayer to release guilt and forgive yourself, before apologizing to them.

♥ Before making love; circling your hips and placing your hands all over your body, to arouse and ready yourself for action.

No matter when or how you dance, the movement releases stress and transports you into a wilder, freer, more magical, and sexier expression of self. Deep in movement, **you think less and feel more**—and this is essential for tuning in and turning up your sensuality! Dancing is an opportunity to appreciate your beautiful post-baby body and celebrate your luscious curves and perfect imperfections: the broad strength of your shoulders, the desirable sway of your hips, the touchable softness of your belly. This is a moment to love and worship yourself, to let the exhaustion and agitation wash away.

. . . .

You're just one dance away from feeling happier, sexier,
and more passionate about yourself.

. . . .

Every day can feel orgasmic when you give yourself permission to own your Mojo, to move like yourself and to love yourself in your own skin. So, let's put on our dancing shoes and get to it!

It's time to use the power of dance to tune into your post-baby body, Mama—to swirl, sway, and shimmy your way into a happier, sexier, and less stressed you. Here are a few suggestions to get you started:

1. Take Five

Whenever you feel tired, irritated, worried, stressed, or on the verge of a mommy meltdown, take a five-minute Mommy Mojo Dance Break. Whenever you find yourself getting lost in the vortex of Facebook feeds and getting caught in the comparison trap about how other moms appear to be doing better than you are, DANCE. Whenever you're feeling like your sex drive is nowhere to be found, turn up the music and DANCE! A dance break unloads the burdens of motherhood and turns down the volume on your inner critic. By moving your body, you have a chance to change how you feel in an instant.

To own your dance break, let everyone know that mommy needs a time-out. Turn on something educational and entertaining for the kids so they don't interrupt you (Tip: screen time is your friend here). Lock your door, dim the lights, and turn on music that moves you. Dress up in something sultry or strip down to a bralette and boy shorts. Plant yourself in front of a full-length mirror *and move*. Dance in a way that feels like a release in that moment: slow and sultry, wild and fast, modern and melancholic, or passionate and provocative. Just move the way YOU want to move, and let it feel natural.

As you dance, drink in your curves. This is YOU. This is YOUR BODY. Every mark tells a story, where your body stretched to grow your child, where your body was cut to birth your child. Your breasts may not be as perky or full these days . . . *because they fed another human being*! Stop the criticism and turn down any negativity that starts to bubble up. Don't let judgment into this sacred space—just dance into yourself, feeling every rise and fall of the melody in your body, telling yourself just how gorgeous you are with every turn. Recognize what your body has done for you and pose the question, *How sensually can I move, right here, right now?* Then, drop even more deeply into yourself.

Acknowledge any worries, fears, guilt, frustration, or rage that may arise, and let it all flow out of you to create space for fresh feelings to rush in. If you feel silly, *laugh*! If you feel like crying, *go right ahead*. If you want to scream, *do it*.

Once you're in the flow, start running your hands over your body with a feather-light touch. Arch your back, circle your hips slowly from side to side, give your booty a playful smack while you lovingly gaze at yourself in the mirror. Touch your breasts and your stomach, and run your hands through your hair. This is *your* body, so love it right up!

Most of all, dance like YOU. Dance to become more fully, completely YOU. Don't worry about "acting sexy." You don't have to act. You simply ARE. Your authenticity as a woman and dedication as a mother is what's sexy. And if you stumble or lose the rhythm as you move, well, that's all part of it.

Your Mission: Take a Mommy Mojo Dance Break every day for one week. Dance before breakfast, after work, before a parent-teacher conference, on a morning where the baby was up all night, or before you plan on having sex with your spouse. Tune in to how you're feeling before and after you dance, and pause to notice any changes in your body confidence and sensuality. Can you bring the hotness and presence you're igniting through dance into the rest of your day?

Note: Dancing might just ignite your Mojo too, and maybe even evolve into a Solo Session. If you feel an urge, act on it!

Bonus: Music is the magic that'll get your Mojo moving! You can access my favorite Sexy Dance Break playlists at www. DanaBMyers.com/resources.

2. Shake What Your Mama Gave You . . . *with Other Women in the Room*!

When you dance, you have an opportunity to physically process the emotions you experience as a mother: the sweet victories and desperate longings, the exhaustion, joy, and frustration . . . all of it! A dance class in a group setting is one of the most cathartic ways to do just that.

There are so many kinds of dance to try as well; you don't have to stick to any one type. Styles like pole dancing and burlesque can create a sense of empowered, erotic ownership of your body, and tango and modern dance can help you express yourself in ways you never imagined. Each style of dance can help you to discover something new about yourself, uncovering another aspect of your sensuality and providing a unique release.

Now it's your turn. Your homework is to research a dance class that excites you—and to find the time in your schedule to get yourself there. If you're nervous about shaking your booty in front of a room filled with strangers, start with something simple like Zumba or basic hip-hop. Or if you're just raring to go, opt for a super juicy class like Afro-Caribbean dance or Kizomba, pushing you past your comfort zone. Go forth on your own, or even enlist a few members of your Mom Tribe to share the transformative experience with you. Taking dance classes with your mom friends surrounds you with all that divine feminine energy, which feels electric, inspiring, and motivating. But whether it's friends or strangers, when you dance together, you purge together, shed your fears, and rev up each other's sensuality.

Your Mission: Commit to two dance classes, or dance-related fitness classes, per month. If budget is an issue, check out the internet for deals. ClassPass.com is a great place to start!

And after you hit the dance floor . . .

3. Increase Your Sensual Strength with Kegels

Okay, so all this dancing is going to improve your mood, fire up your femininity, and inspire some serious self-expression. And once you become a regular dance machine, you'll even start to tone your abs and lift your tush. Dance is also an opportunity to focus on increasing your *sensual strength,* aka the *strength of your pelvic floor.* If you've ever experienced leakage while you're dancing or working out, this tip is for you!

Strong pelvic floor muscles (also called pubococcygeus muscles, or PC muscles for short) are important for women for many reasons. A strong pelvic floor can help boost your orgasms, both in intensity and frequency. That's because squeezing these muscles increases blood flow and improves the muscle tone in your lady parts, which can increase pleasurable sensations. Consistent toning of the PC muscles is what holds your bladder and uterus where they need to be. Since childbearing and birthing causes a lot of stress on these organs (not to mention your vagina!), regular Kegels will help to restrengthen these areas.

Here's how to Kegel like a pro:
Once you're all warmed up after your at-home dance break, or even during a water break at that pole class, give your PC muscles some loving attention with a few focused squeezes.

1. Find your orgasm muscles.

Next time you're peeing, stop yourself midstream—the muscles that stop the flow are your PC muscles, and they are also responsible for the contractions you feel as you orgasm. Once you've got that down, squeeze and lift the muscles in your lower abdomen for additional toning. Once you have the motion down pat, *don't* make a habit of doing it while you pee, since doing so can actually weaken the muscles over time.

2. Squeeze and release.

Hold one Kegel for three seconds, followed by a three-second rest. Repeat ten times for one set. *Do three sets every day, after your dance break.* Remember to breathe!

3. Step it up a notch.

Once three-second holds become easier, switch it to four-second holds and four-second rests, and so on and so forth. As you get stronger, try squeezing and releasing to the beat of the music that's playing during your at-home dance party or group class.

Don't get disheartened if you feel weak when you're first starting out. With practice, you'll soon be amazed at your increased strength and control and will be a Kegel pro in no time.

NEVER MISS A CHANCE TO DANCE

Dance today. Dance tomorrow. And Kegel every damn day while you're at it! Observe how dance moves you from feeling stuck or down to feeling lit up from the inside out. Notice how as you strengthen your pelvic floor from your Kegel exercises how much more sensually empowered and connected your whole body feels.

Once you've done your five-minute Dance Break or taken your first class, and completed your first successful round of Kegel exercises, jot down your thoughts on how it all went.

At what moment in your day did you take a dance break or take a class? How were you feeling before dancing?

_____

_____

_____

_____

_____

What music did you play? Was there a particular song that got you tuned into the experience?

_____

_____

_____

_____

_____

How did dancing make you feel? Sensual, sexy, and free? What other emotions did it reveal and/or heal?

_____

_____

_____

_____

_____

_____

How did you incorporate your Kegel exercises into the experience? How'd that go?

_____

_____

_____

_____

_____

_____

Let's Talk about Sex, Baby

I ONCE MENTORED A MARRIED couple who were going through a prolonged dry spell in their sex life. Naturally, the topic of *talking about sex* came up. Here's how that conversation went:

Her: Ugh. I don't want to talk about sex with him anymore.

Me: Well, why not? What do the conversations sound like?

Her: It's always the same. He says, *When can we have sex? We haven't had sex in five days. Why don't you want to have sex anymore? Can we have sex now? I need sex! We don't have enough sex since having kids.* There's nothing fun about that conversation—all it does is put pressure, expectations, and unnecessary blame on me. The more we talk like this, the less I want to have sex with him.

They were stuck in a cycle of one-sided conversations about the lack of sex in their life—and it was doing nothing but building up more resistance to breaking the spell. As a couple, they weren't coming together in an exploratory discourse of how they could reignite the spark. And you know what? This isn't uncommon. So many couples with kids fall into a pattern of only talking about the shortages in their sex life. Not exactly a sexy conversation!

So I shared a simple communication process with her that would radically change the way she and her husband approached their conversations about sex. It shifted their discussion from what was lacking to what was possible, from his neediness to his desire for her. It was an empowering breakthrough for them, and it helped to take some of the pressure off. I'm pretty sure it was some of the most productive advice I've ever given.

Now, get ready Mama . . . it's your turn.

THE TOOL:
COMMUNICATE YOUR DESIRES

Today you're going to talk about sex with your spouse or partner. As you start finding your way back together in the bedroom with the Sexy Sessions, you also need to get real and raw about what it is you both desire from your sex life. Communicating your needs and desires to your partner, and hearing theirs in return, is essential to feeling satisfied—and to cocreating the fulfilling sex life and authentic intimacy you both deserve.

No longer will your uncomfortable sex conversations be just about the *lack of action* in your relationship. It's time to discuss the actual sex you're having, and the wide range of options that exist to improve it. No more will the conversation spiral into a painful pattern of expectation, resistance, and blame. Today, you'll openly explore the details of your sensual desires with one another and expand your capacity to communicate your needs in a loving, even flirtatious, manner. The key is to leave shyness and judgment at the door and transform old communication conflict into an openhearted discussion.

The secret to great sex begins in the mind, and then it matures and evolves through effective communication. Good sexual communication will help you create the spicy sex life and rich connection you want *and* deserve, but let's face it: sometimes it's hard to find the words—and then figure out how to use them.

Keep in mind that nerves are normal! Even someone who's well versed in disclosing their deepest desires gets tongue-tied from time to time. So take a deep breath and have some patience with yourself—soon enough you'll be connecting in ways you never could have imagined.

Getting Comfortable with the Conversation

If you and your partner haven't been engaging regularly in open and loving sex communication, it's going to feel a little awkward at first. But if you never honestly talk about what you want and need more of, you'll simply never get it! If you never give your partner the opportunity to share his desires, you're keeping yourself in the dark, unable to fulfill his needs, too. Being willing and vulnerable enough to engage in open sex talk will go a long way in building trust between you and your partner; the more trust you build, the deeper your sexual explorations.

But, let's be clear: You're not here to revert back to how sex used to be before you had kids. The point is to work together with your partner to discuss and learn what feels both exciting and satisfying *today,* and to become reacquainted with one another's desires and preferences as lovers (*not* just as parents).

Now, let's start building those sexy communication skills with a journaling exercise about your sex life.

STEP 1: Sex Life Satisfaction—Time to Check In

The first step to improving your postpartum sexual communication is to journal about your own Sex Life Satisfaction. Use the blank spaces below to write about what's really working in your sex life right now, and what you'd like to change up. Make a copy of these questions and ask your partner to do the same. Afterward, you'll sit down together to share your thoughts with each other.

What's Great?

What feels good in your sex life *right now?* Are you satisfied with the frequency of your sexual activity together? The playfulness of your encounters? The intensity of your orgasms? The go-to positions you adore? What else?

_____

_____

_____

_____

What Could Be Better?

What sexual challenges stand in the way of having better sex? Are your sex drives out of sync? Does the expectation your partner places on you turn you off? Are you unfulfilled by defaulting to the same positions every time you make love? Are you struggling to reach orgasm because your partner's touch is too intense, or too soft? Do you wish that your lover would initiate sex more often? Do you crave more affection outside the bedroom? Would you like to bring in sex toys to enhance your pleasure? Do you no longer enjoy the feeling of your breasts being kissed, now that you've breastfed? Does the position you used to love before you gave birth now cause you discomfort? What else? Don't be shy. Now is the time to honor your truth.

_____

_____

_____

_____

Note: Consider how you could phrase your answers in a *positive, proactive way.* For example, instead of saying, *"I'm so bored with the same positions every time we have sex,"* you could say, *"Sex could be better if we try some new positions during our next Session."*

What's one specific sexual request you'd like to ask of your partner? This might be anything from having sex in a new location, more passionate kissing, or testing out a slower pace than usual during intercourse. These creative ideas will make it easier to navigate the previous question.

_____

_____

_____

What kind of "sexual energy" would you like to play with?
This might sound something like . . . *I want to explore rougher play for our sex to feel more electric. Or, I want softer, more romantic sex. Or, I want him to toss me on the bed, like he's the strongest man on earth. Or, I want sex to feel more sacred between us, like a prayer.*

How could you cocreate a sex life that feels exciting and compassionate? One that can continue to evolve for the next ten, twenty, thirty, forty years?
It might look like this: *We can talk more often about what's positive, instead of complaining about what's missing. Or, we could plan a "sex date" once a month, every month, no excuses, for the rest of our lives! Or, we can commit to approaching our sex life as a fun adventure, where each of us brings new ideas to the table, taking turns being in charge.*

STEP 2: Opening Up the Lines of Communication with Your Lover
The next step is translating your answers into a loving, sexual discussion.

First, choose the right time and place to have the conversation—and that right time and place is *not* when you're naked in the bedroom, nor is it before, during, or immediately after sex. It's not when he's made a move and you've just turned him down, or when you've just lost your temper at the kids or plopped onto the bed in a heap of exhaustion at the end of the day. All are too vulnerable a space for you and your mate. Instead, bring it up when you're both relaxed and free from distractions.

Next, break the ice by asking and answering the following list of suggestive—but fun—sex questions. These conversation starters will ignite a sense of flirtation and ease you into talking about your sex life in a more serious way. Think of them like a warm-up.

Bringing Sexy Back: A Warm-Up Couples Q&A

♥ What do you remember about the first time we had sex?
♥ What's your favorite position?
♥ What's the naughtiest thought you've ever had about me?
♥ What's the most memorable sex we've ever had?
♥ Where do you want to have sex that we haven't before?
♥ If you named your privates, what would you call it?
♥ What's your favorite spot to be kissed?
♥ What sounds more exciting: ice cubes or warming massage oil?
♥ Have you ever had a sexy dream about me? Describe it.
♥ What do I do that turns you on the most—past or present?
♥ *Should we just stop talking and have sex right now?*

Note: If these flirtatious questions have sparked some desire, then please, dive into whatever kind of sexy time feels right. You can always return to the conversation after your bodies are lit up with pleasure.

THE REAL SEX TALK: Discussion Dos and Don'ts

Now that you're warmed up, it's time to broach the Sex Life Satisfaction Q&As you journaled about. Touch your partner and allow time to get physically comfortable with each other, then take turns sharing your answers to all of the questions, one by one. Try not to interrupt one another. Many people are hesitant to reveal their deepest sexual thoughts and desires out of fear of rejection or ridicule. So be patient, and listen without judgment so your partner feels free to be an equal player in the discussion. Ask that they do the same.

When speaking honestly about your thoughts on *What Could Be Better,* try to be mindful to lead with positive affirmations. Remember: You can't compliment your partner too much or too often during this conversation. After all, this is a sensitive subject and it's important to be conscious of how you address anything you might dislike without bruising your partner's ego.

One simple way to do this is to avoid using the word "but."

For example, you could address the first two questions like this: "Babe, I love the way we (insert answer from *What's Great*), because it makes me feel like you know my body so well, **AND** I want to (insert positive suggestion from *What Could Be Better*).

Avoid saying something like, "I love how I orgasm when I'm on top, **BUT** I'd like to try some new positions, too."

It's a subtle difference in word choices, and while the second example is just as honest as the first, it's laced with criticism. When you turn a phrase with "but," it negates the positive, kind words that came before it.

On addressing specific dislikes . . .

With the approach I just mentioned, it's easy to steer your partner away from what you don't want, and toward more of what you do want. However, if you feel you must specifically address a sexual dislike, such as a move your lover repeatedly does that is causing you discomfort, you could say something like: *"Babe, I love how I orgasm on top, however this (insert particular move) we do is no longer giving me pleasure. I'd love to try (insert alternative) next time we make love. Are you up for it?"*

By using the phrase "we do" instead of "you do," you avoid placing blame and wounding his ego, while showing him that you want to work together to improve your sexual satisfaction.

Remember, these honest conversations can be tough, but the truth will set you free. Being honest is what will break you out of the rut; it's what creates space for intimate growth in your relationship. Be prepared to hear your partner's truth too, which might sound something like, *"It's hard to feel inspired to make a move on you when you always seem irritated with me,"* or *"I've gotten used to you saying no to me, which makes me not want to try at all."*

Continue talking through all the questions with love, understanding, enthusiasm, and curiosity.

Okay, so where do you go from here?

Now that you've spoken your sexual truths, know that you don't have to fix every concern, or immediately fulfill every desire that was spoken— now *or ever.* The exercise is simply to talk about the potential for growth within your sex life and relationship, instead of only focusing on what's lacking.

Just because you've *started* talking about sex here doesn't mean you should stop! Continue the conversation, because practice makes perfect.

The more you talk about sex and your mutual goals for a passionate, satisfying sensual connection, the easier the conversation will become. The more you talk, the more you give yourselves the opportunity to discover solutions *together*.

A final word: talk like humans who love each other!

Whether you're talking about sex, money, or groceries, please remember to talk to one another like *humans who love and respect each other*. It's easy to be defensive, accusatory, short-tempered, and stubborn but always make an effort to communicate with your spouse with loving kindness and respect.

The Long Love Engagement A Sexy Session

B Y THE TIME OUR firstborn was eight months old, the Quickie had resurrected our sex life. It felt like a small miracle, like I was winning at this whole married-with-children sex life thing. But there was still something missing.

It was a Friday night around nine o'clock, and I'd finally gotten the baby to sleep after an epic breastfeeding session. I was ravenous, but despite my hunger I decided to stoke my sexual appetite instead with a Quickie. So I grabbed my husband, pulled him into the hot tub, and we started making love. In my peripheral vision, I caught a glimpse of the Chinese takeout sitting on my kitchen counter. *I could practically taste the sesame chicken.* I felt his intensity building, the finish line was in sight, the crispy spring rolls were calling my name! But then . . . he asked to switch locations. *Would I like to move into the bedroom? Change positions? Grab a sex toy?* He wanted to keep going, to have more fun. The Chinese food was the furthest thing from his mind.

"I'm hungry and I'm tired," I said with a sigh. He asked again, but this time I actually rolled my eyes. "Forget it," he said. "Go eat and sleep." I was still a new mom after all, and naturally all I wanted was to eat and sleep! Wasn't that normal? Wasn't the Quickie enough at this point in our parenting journey? The short answer: No.

We talked it out over takeout, and he said he understood where I was coming from, but he still wanted and needed more from our sex life, both emotionally and physically. He shared how much he missed long, leisurely sexcapades, where we took time for sensual exploration—not just a quick release or an item checked off on our relationship to-do list. He wanted to know that I still desired him, that even though we were now exhausted parents I wasn't just going through the motions to please him.

No matter how tired or hungry I was, I heard him. We had to take more time in the bedroom again and find our way back to each other—to create space for exciting sexual exploration and remember why we fell in love in the first place and started a family. And so, we brought the sexy back with the Long Love Engagement, one of the most important elements of the Mommy Mojo Makeover.

Sexy Session #3: The Long Love Engagement

After that hot tub episode, we met and made love for at least thirty minutes, once a week, *every* week. We played, we explored, we pleasured each other. Sometimes it felt natural, and other times like a chore. But no matter what, we prioritized our physical connection. We followed through on that renewed commitment we'd made to each other as husband and wife and partners in parenting—but, most of all, as lovers.

Now it's your turn. With the Long Love Engagement, **you'll take thirty minutes to rediscover making out, dive back into creative foreplay, try new positions, and still have time left over for**

postcoital cuddling. This is your opportunity to sensually pamper and appreciate each other, and to dramatically increase the amount of touch you share with one another. It's your opportunity to have some fun with toys if you'd like, and slowly build up to big, beautiful orgasms. I want you to move intentionally and feel everything - the good, the bad, and even the awkward.

Open your heart and dare to be vulnerable. Rekindling the physical and emotional connection with your partner with a Long Love Engagement will help you rediscover and redefine what quality sex looks and feels like to you both.

. . . .

Deepen your connection and rekindle desire
with the Long Love Engagement!

. . . .

But I don't have the time! I don't have the passion or desire! That's okay. You may feel so sexually disconnected from your partner that a long, exploratory romp in the bedroom seems impossible. Don't worry. The main goal is to set aside about thirty minutes for sensual time, creating an opportunity to reconnect in a deeper way. In other words: to have more than just a Quickie!

YOUR MISSION: HAVE A THIRTY-MINUTE LOVE SESSION

In order to tackle this sexy beast of a Session, here are some of my favorite tips to help you plan and follow through with the Long Love Session:

1. MAKE A DATE AND STICK TO IT (NO EXCUSES!)

Talk to your partner and plan your Session together, deciding on a time when you'll both feel energized and inspired to actually follow through. Perhaps it's when the kids are napping or go to bed early, or maybe when they're at a friend's house for dinner. Try to plan for a window when you can both step away from your responsibilities and meet for an afternoon or evening delight while no one is at home. I've found it helpful to plan a Long Love Engagement in the daytime—even in the morning—before you have a chance to exhaust yourself. Once you've made your date, put it in your calendars. Your partner will be thrilled you initiated this idea, and you'll feel empowered you took the reigns to get the ball rolling.

Planning lovemaking may seem like a drag, since it seems to take the spontaneity out of sex. For most of us, there was probably a time when sex was effortless and didn't require scheduling. But trust me, Mamas, if we didn't plan sex—especially when kids are under five—most couples would never have it. Think of it as a joint effort to bring passion and desire back to your sex life. I promise that as you build momentum with the planned Sessions in this book, spontaneous sex will inevitably return to your love life.

2. STAY CURIOUS . . . AND STAY PRESENT

Once you've scheduled your Session, it's time to show up and get down to business. But I mean *really* show up, by being fully present in mind and body. If your plan is to have sex at night after the kids are down, I invite you to take fifteen minutes to yourself to get centered. Breathe, take a quick bath, meditate, stretch, have a glass of wine, maybe even dance a little. Ask your partner to prep dinner so that it'll be ready when your Session is done. These fifteen minutes of me-time are critical to showing up for your Session in a relaxed, revitalized way. Going straight from kiddie bedtimes to sexy time is a big no-no. You won't feel patient, and you most certainly won't feel enthusiastic. You need to take the time to decompress from the chaos of the day and ease into a more sensual state. Got that? Good.

Put on some music and begin your Long Love Session by breathing together and gazing into one another's eyes, caressing each other's faces, and kissing for longer than you usually do. Or, step into a hot shower and lather up each other's bodies with deliciously-scented soap. However you choose to begin, simply be present together. You may feel some resistance here, especially if it's been awhile since you last had sex or if you hear a peep on the baby monitor. Try to relax and stay open, freeing your mind from what's on your to-do list, and letting go of any frustrations or criticisms you may be feeling toward your partner. Soften your heart. Then, soften up even more! Remember you *love this person.* Allow yourself to be curious about what pleasure might await you.

If you start this Sexy Session and your mind is racing, you feel uneasy about the time commitment, or if it's simply been ages since you've made love like this, try this mental trick to help you relax:

As your partner kisses you, silently repeat in your mind, *"I welcome your kiss."*

As he touches you, *"I welcome your touch."*

And so on and so forth.

As you calm your mind with these silent mantras, you'll find that your body will calm down too. Your goal is simply to stay engaged with your partner for thirty minutes (or more!), and these miracle mantras can help get you there.

3. CHANNEL YOUR INNER EXPLORER

Many moms at my workshops tell me that the average amount of time their sexual encounters take from start to finish is ten minutes. So in order to stretch your Long Love Session to thirty minutes, try exploring a variety of sensual pleasures like dancing with each other, massage, oral exploration, penetration, kissing, new positions, taking a short break, incorporating a couples' vibrator, manual stimulation, etc. Then, simply repeat what feels good.

Be sure to communicate. Ask each other questions like, *Does that feel good? How would you like me to touch you? Can I nibble on you here? Would you like to try . . . ?* The more you talk during sex, the more your partner will do the same.

After this exploratory sensual time together, you should feel ready to climax. *But maybe not.* Don't get hung up on having a big, beautiful orgasm, as this Session is more about reconnecting sensually without pressure or expectation. It might feel refreshing and surprisingly easy, or it may be awkward and clumsy. The point is to just get it going again! However, if you feel you *can* orgasm, I encourage you to use whatever positions, props, and toys you need to get there. Bonus: If you do, you'll release oxytocin, a key "love hormone" linked with all kinds of feel-good emotions like trust, empathy, and bonding.

4. CELEBRATE THE SEX YOU JUST HAD

Congrats, you did it! You set a sex date and followed through. Perhaps it was the first Long Love Session you've had in weeks, months, or even years. Now, take a moment to seal in the magic you just created together with some postcoital pillow talk.

Tell each other what felt great and why. Something like, "Babe, I feel amazing after that orgasm. What you did with your hands made me see stars . . . I'm so glad we did that!" Then, ask what really worked for him. Do this all while maintaining loving physical contact. While it may seem odd, congratulating yourselves and celebrating the sex you just had will go miles toward boosting intimacy and strengthening your bond as lovers. Plus, it's way more fun than talking about bedtimes and baby poop.

5. GET YOUR NEXT SESSION ON THE CALENDAR

Because your body and mind are freshly lit up with pleasure, planning your next Session immediately should feel like a joy—not a chore. It's also a perfect opportunity to express a sensual desire you'd like to fulfill with the one you love. You might say something like, "That felt so good! Next time I'd love to try this position/toy/etc. So, how's Thursday morning for you, babe?"

Whatever you do, don't skip over these last two steps. It's this approach that makes scheduled sex a beautiful, communicative, passionate celebration, all while creating genuine anticipation for your next Session together. You'll have a specific date and time to look

---

Note: I shared my hot tub story to remind you that men have strong emotional needs too, and that it's not always just about wanting pure physical pleasure. You *both* need the Long Love Session to feel desired, and to explore with each other while expressing yourselves sexually. Creating long-term passion after having kids requires both players to recommit to intimacy and each other—over and over, again and again. Connecting through a Long Love Session will make you stronger as a couple, and isn't that what you both want?

forward to, fantasize about, and mentally prepare for. Planning and following through also builds trust around sex in your relationship—and that faith is the glue that binds you in parenthood and marriage.

With the Long Love Session, sex will start to feel like something you *get* to do, rather than something you *have* to do. And trust me, there's a lot more sex to be had in the coming parts, so stay tuned!

YOUR SEXY SESSIONS JOURNAL: As with all your Sexy Sessions, it's time to reflect. Take a moment to recall your Long Love Session with your spouse and journal your thoughts, free-form or by answering these questions:

1. How would you describe your Long Love Session?

_____

_____

_____

_____

_____

2. What was your process of planning like with your spouse? How was your communication?

_____

_____

_____

_____

_____

3. Before you began, did you take time to relax into a sensual state of being? If so, how?

_____

_____

_____

_____

_____

_____

_____

4. What sensations felt most pleasurable and intimate? Or was there any awkwardness or disconnection?

_____

_____

_____

_____

_____

_____

5. Did you celebrate afterward with pillow talk? What did you each say to each other?

_____

_____

_____

_____

_____

6. Did you plan your next Session? For when?

_____

_____

_____

_____

_____

_____

_____

Go Wild with Your Mom Tribe

MOTHERHOOD IS MAGICAL, and it is without a doubt the most meaningful experience of my life. And yet, motherhood is *hard.* It's often messy, confusing, and isolating. Sometimes I feel like a Supermom capable of juggling it all, and other times I become so overwhelmed that I wonder how I'll get through the day.

But without fail, a mama friend is always there to comfort me. The phone rings or a text comes in and the simple phrase, "you doin' okay?" calms me every time. I talk and cry it out—getting it all off my chest. I remember that *I am not alone;* that I am supported.

This is the nourishing power of a Mom Tribe, the mothers in my life whom I can talk to about sippy cups and sex, successes and self-doubt. My Mom Tribe is made up of women I can *go deep* with, baring my truest self without pretense—and knowing I'll be received without judgment.

The women in my Mom Tribe remind one another, every single day, that we don't have to be perfect. We talk endlessly until we've uncovered the lessons and gifts hidden in our epic mom-fails. We take each other's kids to gymnastics and borrow outfits from our closets. We bring breakfast muffins and hold each other up over freshly brewed coffee. This is all part of our pact: our sacred, supportive agreement as a Mom Tribe.

Go Wild with Your Mom Tribe

But, above all, the best part about our pact as a Mom Tribe is our commitment to having raucous fun together. We plan boozy moms' nights out and dance with abandon together. We play hooky after the school drop-off and go out exploring in nature. We Pop-Out to art openings and let daddy feed and put the kids to bed. We go to twerking classes and learn to shake our thighs in ways we never thought possible. There are our *Wild Woman Outings,* and they serve as a creative outlet to sensually express ourselves, free from our roles and responsibilities as mothers. Our only task is to liberate ourselves with wild abandon; focused solely on having FUN. We make them happen at least once a month, *every* month, no excuses.

I've noticed in my workshops that many moms will confess that the time spent with their mom friends has been reduced to sideline chats on the field or noisy playdates where they're constantly being interrupted. They say there's just not enough time nor budget for a wild moms' night out. Some will even admit that they don't feel like they have *permission* . . . as though their "wild days" are over now that they're moms.

If that sounds all too familiar then let me remind you that you do have permission. In fact it is essential to your Mommy Mojo Makeover.

The wild ways in which you can connect on a deeper level with your Mom Tribe are endless: a riotous night at the bar, a frisky adult-themed shopping party, a private pole-dancing lesson, or even a champagne-fueled drawing class with a handsome naked male model.

But I want to share one idea in particular that has proven to be one of the most liberating and pleasurable experiences for my Mom Tribe: **A Wild Woman Photo Shoot.** This is a four-hour outing that leaves every single mama in the party feeling lit up, creative, and body confident, with a sense of unleashed freedom that resonates for *days, weeks, even months afterward.*

. . . .

In this Wild Woman Outing, every mama will feel celebrated for the sexy, playful, powerful, and unique woman that she is.

. . . .

THE EXPERIENCE:
THE WILD WOMAN PHOTO SHOOT

YOUR MISSION: Take the initiative and lead a Wild Woman Photo Shoot. Email your girls, choose a date, pick your props, and get your cameras ready. The time has come to unleash the Wild Woman within . . . and to do so together!

Here are the six short and simple steps for creating a Wild Woman Photo Shoot of your own:

Step 1: Gather Your Tribe
Choose a time to gather with your Mom Tribe. For example, right after school drop-off, say 9:00 a.m.—this way, no one needs to book a sitter. Ask if anyone has a love for photography and would like to be the designated photographer, otherwise you can all collectively snap pictures

with your phones. Brainstorm locations and themes in advance (think Rock and Roll, Nature Goddess, Boudoir, etc.), and tell everyone to bring a bag of outfits, accessories, and props (like scarves, feathers, gloves, heels), and their makeup bags, too.

Step 2: Transform Together

Upon arrival, spend about forty-five minutes getting ready *together*. Put on music, play with makeup, dress each other up, swap accessories, and compliment each other with abundant enthusiasm. It's like old-school times when getting ready together was just the norm. Drink coffee, indulge in pastries, even whip up a pitcher of mimosas. Start snapping photos during the primping hour.

Step 3: Lights, Camera, Action!

Head to your photo shoot location. It might be somewhere in nature: a tranquil park, a mystical forest, a flowing stream. Or the city: a busy square, a bustling public park, a sexy street with shops and attractions. Or, keep it simple and hang out in your backyard or a well-lit room in your home. Turn on some music and start taking pictures! Explore posed or candid shots as a group, and then try couples, trios, and solos. It may feel awkward at first, but the more you snap, the looser and more flowing the session will become. Moving through any nervousness will only strengthen everyone's feminine confidence. As you get into the flow, initiate topics of conversation that don't relate to your kids. Talk about sex, your childhood, spirituality, and the future . . . and see how that conversation shapes and shifts everyone's moods and expressions. Or, just crack jokes and laugh together!

Step 4: Play with Props

Bust out the props and get creative with them. Have everyone wave a scarf in the wind, or cross their legs while wearing heels. Dance or strike a yoga pose. Make ridiculous, serious, or sexy faces. Hug each other. Remember to compliment one another's bodies and beauty. You'll start to see a different aspect of your friends' personalities emerge—that's their *inner Wild Woman*. Feel the exhilaration building. As a finale to the shoot, seek out one last, unexplored location: a new tree to climb, a busy street corner, a beautiful nook in the house.

Step 5: Finish with a Tribe Circle

Stand together in a circle and take turns describing how you feel using words like *empowered, sensual, intelligent, rock star, ballsy, radiant, free, mysterious, feminine, turned on.*

Step 6: Sharing Is Caring

Once the group's energy starts to wane, gather back at the house to sit and chat about the experience as you huddle around the cameras to check out all your amazing photos. In advance, create a private shared album and be sure everyone knows how to upload their best shots. If budget allows, consider making mini photo albums for everyone as a memento— a treasured reminder of the magic and beauty you've created together.

But Will It Work? Here's Why Mamas Need to Go Wild:

Although it may seem like a simple event, the effects of a Wild Woman Photo Shoot are radical—healing—even, as each mama peels back the layers of the perfectly put together mother and unleashes the playful, sensual woman inside for the camera to capture and the Mom Tribe to witness.

The Wild Woman Photo Shoot is like a secret gathering that carries a slight sense of danger, creativity, and sensual expression as you play dress-up and run wild—expressing yourselves and capturing it all on film. It's an unusual and amazing experience that reminds each of you how bold, sexy, and fun you truly are.

All too often, moms are too wrapped up in a tightly controlled state of being, and a wild experience can instantly infuse our existence with more pleasure and fun. Wild Woman Outings and photo shoots are dramatic departures from what we *usually* do together as moms, and that alone will create a renewed sense of freedom and vitality within you, as well as a deepening of the bonds within your Mom Tribe.

Sex Up Your Space

BEFORE HAVING CHILDREN, I was one of those women who was *certain* that our home would NEVER be overrun by toys and baby bouncers, and riddled with all things plastic.

Ha! How wrong I was.

Once our kids arrived, the common spaces of our home fell into a fast decline. What was once a fairly stylish living room quickly became an explosion of kid things. The kitchen? Forget it. Overrun by sippy cups, Mickey Mouse plates, high chairs, and walkers. For a while, I was able to stop the flow of plastic crap from seeping into our bedroom—the last bastion of grown-up privacy we had left to ourselves.

But slowly, no matter how hard I tried, the kid mess crept into our bedroom, too. First it was breast pump accessories on the night-stand (a noticeable shift from massage oils and feather ticklers). Then, stuffed animals on the bed, misplaced binkies crammed into every nook, toy school buses on the floor, and stacks of books on every surface.

Our bedroom had transformed from being a sanctuary of erotic inspiration and oasis for seduction to a constant reminder of . . . well . . . parenthood. And as much as I truly cherish our life as a family, it turns out that a cluttered, kid-invaded bedroom doesn't make for much of a love nest.

My husband and I made a commitment to reclaim our bedroom as a boudoir: a space to call our own—a sensual retreat where we could frolic freely as a twosome once more. We cleared out the clutter, put away all the kid stuff, and sprinkled a few spicy touches to turn us back on. It didn't take much time or money, yet the small effort made a huge difference in transforming the bedroom back to a sexually stimulating and arousing space. There was a noticeable shift in our moods when we entered the bedroom; a palpable sensual energy had begun to manifest itself once again.

Creating a Sensual Space for Intimacy

It takes effort from all angles to reignite an inspired sex life: self-confidence, communication, and a mutual commitment to the cause, to name a few. But also, we must stimulate all of the senses, in all our environments. Creating a sensual space for intimacy is integral to sparking desire and, ultimately, having a great sex life.

Your bedroom is your Relationship HQ. It's the epicenter where you connect, communicate, and make the magic happen (or where you're trying to make it happen). But let's be realistic: you have kids! The good news is that a "sexy bedroom" doesn't have to look like a bordello or an S&M dungeon. But it shouldn't look like a toy store exploded in there either.

With just a bit of effort, sexing up your space will make you and your partner feel like lovers again, rather than roommates. Follow these simple tips to transform—and maintain—your bedroom into a special place that turns you both on; a tactile sexual playground that inspires your shared sensuality.

. . . .

**Say goodbye to unsexy clutter and
hello to a bedroom that really lights your fire!**

. . . .

YOUR MISSION: GIVE YOUR BEDROOM A MAKEOVER TOGETHER

With your spouse or partner, take an afternoon and evening, or a Saturday morning while the kids are at Grandma's, and do as many of these suggestions as you can. Pour your love into creating a more seductive space to share together, one that inspires you both to feel more relaxed and romantic.

Doing this bedroom makeover together, instead of on your own, is an act that says,

We recognize that desire and lust aren't just going to reappear magically . . . but that we can slowly but surely bring it back to life by working TOGETHER.

Then, stay on top of it. Make your bed every morning, *together*. Flirt and say, *I can't wait to dive back in here with you tonight,* as you fluff the pillows or playfully swat each other with them. This invitation creates anticipation and excitement. Also, make it a point to declutter the room once a week together. If you feel as though your partner is losing the motivation to help you, say something like, *Babe, you know it really turns me on when you pick up after yourself.* From personal experience, Mamas, this simple sentence works like a charm!

It's time to transform your bedroom into a *playroom*—for adults only. These quick fixes will give your bedroom an immediate boost, and many of these sexy upgrades require hardly any time or money at all!

1. Ditch the Clutter and Technology

Your surroundings influence your life and mood—period. A cluttered, messy bedroom will frustrate you to no end, leaving you both feeling claustrophobic and totally unsexy. Make it a practice to put your clothes straight into the hamper or back in the closet—not on the floor or draped over a chair. Throw out old magazines and outdated birthday cards, or put them into a special keepsake box in your closet. Move exercise equipment to another room, and stop "storing things" in corners or under your bed. By clearing away the excess, you're creating mental and physical space for romance. Warning: The digital clutter needs to go too! Remove the screens from your sensual space—smartphones, tablets, and TVs—they are just too great of a distraction from exploring your sensual connection. Now, if you *only* do this one step, I assure you that you will notice a difference in how much sexier, more relaxed, and in tune with your partner you'll feel in the bedroom.

2. Make Your Sensual Space a Kid-, Work-, and In-Law-Free Zone

Jettison any traces of work or domestic responsibilities from your new boudoir; they're just a reminder of all the things you need to do and the stressful week ahead. Hide your to-do lists and keep your laptop in another room. This will help keep your stress levels at bay and your mind more focused on the romantic possibilities at hand. Clear out family photos of anyone who shouldn't be watching you while you have sex—send the pic of your mother-in-law to the den! Kid toys and stuffed animals are a reminder that you're a great parent, but not necessarily a sexy mama. Stow them in their proper place. It's all a distraction from putting your Mojo first, plus stepping on Legos in your lingerie is also a major buzzkill. I'm not suggesting your bedroom becomes a place where your kids aren't invited, but at the very least, you shouldn't be tripping over their toys scattered across the floor. Keep a beautiful woven basket with a lid in the corner and stash a few kid staples in there for those Saturday morning play sessions with mom and dad in bed. Tip: If you co-sleep, do the same for the rooms where you usually go to make love.

3. Switch Up the Furniture

Do what you can to improve the energetic flow of your space. A clear path will make the room feel more comfortable and welcoming—you'll want to linger there longer because it won't feel so erratic. There's nothing sexy about knocking your knees against that chair you've been meaning to move out of the room. Get creative and switch up the floor plan of your furniture: move the bed, shift the dresser, and rehang the mirrors. It'll feel like a new bedroom, fresh with renewed energy and sex appeal.

4. Use Soft Lighting to Flatter and Seduce

The right lighting has the power to create intimacy, warmth, and instant ambiance. If you can, switch over your lamps and overhead fixtures to dimmers. Get a side table lamp shaped with sensual, voluptuous curves. Invest in a set of ten flameless candles—you'll find the warm light enchanting, plus there's no risk of fire. If you and your partner are generally more playful, string up some delicate twinkle lights to add charm and a touch of youthful fantasy.

5. Seek Out Pleasurable Bedding and Pillows

Soft, luscious, plush, heavenly blankets and sheets are wonderful for enveloping your naked body. Silks, good satins, high-quality silk cotton and soft-spun wool (for blankets and throws) feel super sexy. If you're on a budget, I recommend jersey cotton sheets. They're so soft that you'll never wear pajamas to bed again! Search for throw pillows with textures you want to reach out and rub your skin against—perhaps faux fur, lace, or even delicate strips of leather fringe. You want everything on your bed to be inviting, pleasurable, and irresistible to the touch.

6. Set a Sensual Mood with Fragrance

Scent can be a big turn-on in your bedroom, transporting you away from your busy mom life or workday, and into your own personal sexy playground. Light scented candles, burn oils, or set out fragrance sticks—think vanilla, musk, sandalwood, even a hint of cinnamon, or something with a subtle combination of sweet and spicy. If your budget allows, place an arrangement of blooming, fragrant flowers near the bed. If you know that a certain perfume you wear drives your partner wild, try misting your sheets with it and see what unfolds.

7. Keep a Seductive Book on Hand

No matter how sexy your bedroom looks, there's always room for a little extra stimulation to get you in the mood. Keep an anthology of sexy stories or a book of provocative photography on your bedside table. You can look at it on your own and fantasize before a Solo Session, or thumb through it with your lover and discuss what's sexy about each story or photo. In contrast to the Dr. Seuss book your toddler left on the nightstand or that anxiety-inducing parenting book you keep trying to finish, this will be an instant turn-on.

8. Keep Treats Nearby

Have little bites of chocolate in a delicate glass bowl next to the bed: a little bite of dark chocolate can be the perfect follow-up to an incredible orgasm. Also, keep your favorite sex toys, massage oils, and lubricants at arm's reach in your nightstand drawer. Remember: You're turning your bedroom into a playroom, so you're going to need some adults-only toys to have fun with! If you're concerned about little hands finding things they shouldn't, get a storage box for your sex toys—complete with lock and key.

9. Arouse and Energize with Music

Get back into the habit of playing music in the bedroom again. Like lighting, music has the power to immediately transport you into a more seductive mood. Since what makes music sexy is so personal, explore the sounds that turn you on: R&B, samba, ambient, or maybe some rock and roll. Build several seduction playlists full of the songs that get your Mojo firing and then . . . turn it on!

As you begin to reestablish mutual pleasure in your new sensual space, you can incorporate more sexiness into the game by taking a shopping trip together to purchase sexy-but-comfy jammies, soft slippers, and plush lounging robes—things you want to luxuriate in while you're enjoying your new boudoir. It may sound simple, but making over your bedroom and increasing the pleasure you experience in there is an act of sexy self-care as a couple. It's a joint effort that translates into an invitation to talk more, play more, and make more sweet, sensual love.

Bring Back
That Lovin' Feeling

WE JUST FEEL MORE like roommates than lovers . . .

I've heard this statement more times than I can count from moms and dads alike. That natural, flirtatious connection that once existed between you and your partner has faded away. That connection that once said with just a simple glance, *I'm SO into you.*

It breaks my heart that parenting could have this kind of effect on two people who were once so enthusiastically in love. But it can—and it does. Over time it starts to feel like you've become business partners just trying to get through another tough day at the office—with little tyrants testing your patience at every turn.

I know this feeling because I've been there myself.

In the early days of parenting I'll admit that I may have killed our romantic connection. To be more precise, I slaughtered it. As a new mother, I planned every minute of every day around the baby. That kind of rigorous schedule and routine gave me a sense of control in what was an otherwise chaotic transition into motherhood. But looking back now, I realize I'd actually gone off the deep end.

Instead of snuggling on the couch with my man at night, I'd sit at the kitchen table reading sleep-training books. If he tried to kiss me while I was cooking baby food, I'd wave him off, annoyed he was "trying to distract" me from my baby task at hand. Once, he asked me to come outside to look at the stars with him and I outright refused! I shot down a gorgeous offer from my loving husband because I was busy sterilizing a sink full of bottles.

That was my wake-up call moment: my absurd refusal of a romantic proposition.

WTF was I thinking? What had happened to me? What other opportunities was I missing to connect with my husband?

I was a *woman* who'd become *all mother*: all mission, all the time. During my transition into motherhood, I stopped seeing my husband as my lover, my other half, my fuel that helped get me through my day. I was neglecting his affections, his attempts to flirt and be spontaneous. I had removed romance from our daily ritual; I'd lost focus on the *us*.

So I had to figure out how to lighten up and start loving *us* up again. I took a good hard look at the ways I was participating in the de-romancing of our relationship, and I made a conscious effort to bring back that lovin' feeling that brought us together in the first place.

Marriage can be monotonous, and yes, it's easy to lose that amorous edge as the years go by. But you don't want to neglect your *us*, for the sake of the children. You don't want that electric spark between you to fizzle out. Because think about it: your children *will* grow up and leave the house, and then you'll still have *decades* left with your spouse! *Eesh.* Don't we all want a lover to ride into the sunset with? Of course we do! So I'll let you in on a little secret: It starts outside the bedroom with a bit of daily flirtation, romantic inspiration, and conscious connection.

. . . .

Keep passion alive by making
conscious connection a priority.

. . . .

Rehab Your Romance

After years of marriage, flirting isn't so much about seductively licking your lips or throwing down a sexy pickup line. It's when you do something each day to inspire your partner to fall in love with you again and again—and invite them to do the same—creating a reciprocation of positive energy.

It's time to move toward each other again in an effort to say, *Hey, I love you, I'm interested in you, in us. I want to continue building our love story!* Because feeling more like a passionate couple outside the bedroom will go a LONG way to helping you get your groove back *in* the bedroom.

Inspired by my own experience in romance rehab, below are some ideas to help you bring back that lovin' feeling in your relationship.

YOUR MISSION: Choose one or more to try out today to immediately bring back a hint of that lovin' feeling.

1. Kiss More

Have you noticed that you and your spouse kiss much less these days? But the more you kiss your spouse, the more connected your relationship will be. Why? Because it requires you to get in each other's personal space several times a day and is a tool to quickly drop petty annoyances, communicate that you love each other, and show support without speaking a single word. Simply put, a kiss is a connection point.

Try this: Kiss your partner at least ten times every day for a week, and see what happens.

2. Touch Each Other Without Expectation

The same goes for more physical connection. Reach for your partner's hand or arm as you're chatting over breakfast, then go in for a quick hug before you rush the kids to school. Initiate a spontaneous thumb-wrestling match on your way out to the gym, or rest your head on his shoulder as you watch the kids play. If your favorite song comes on, grab him for a quick dance session in the middle of the kitchen, and squeeze him tightly. This kind of physical affection outside the bedroom says, *I want to feel connected to you.*

Note: Many moms say they feel a heavy sense of expectation when their husbands initiate this kind of touch, fearing that it will lead to sex—and maybe they're just too damn tired to participate. I think the issue is that moms can feel like they've had too much touch as is! There's an abundance of hugs and kisses, which fills you up with positive physical affection, as well as a long day of tugs and pulls upon our every limb, which can start to make a mama feel as though her body is not her own. And so by the end of the day, she's probably had enough.

The next time your partner comes up from behind you and nuzzles your neck the minute the kids have gone down for bed, you may cringe and think, *Oh no. If I respond and reciprocate, he'll think I want to have sex.* Even though a long, warm hug might feel lovely, you wiggle out of his embrace, muttering something about the next thing you have to do.

If this is the case, try this: Make a commitment with your partner to touch *more* throughout the day, *without* the expectation that things will go further. It may take time for him to fully grasp this concept, and for you to learn to trust and welcome his touch. Next time he goes in for an embrace and your inner voice shouts "No!"—pause and breathe, Mama. Fight the urge to flee, even if you have something to do or somewhere to be. Lean into his touch, feel your energies connect, and reciprocate the embrace with enthusiasm. If he forgets about your commitment and attempts to move into sex, remind him how you agreed to practice touch without expectation. If that feels too robotic, you could say something like, "Mmm, that embrace feels so good, babe, but I'm going to take a rain check on sex right now. I've got some other things planned. Can we wait until I can give you my full atten-tion?" Easy enough, right?

3. Make a Surprise Gesture

An unprompted romantic act can start as simple as bringing home a bottle of his favorite whiskey or writing a love note he discovers in his briefcase at work. Even better, record a voice memo on his phone recounting your favorite date or telling him in detail what you love about him. (Tip: Be sure to set an alarm for him that says, "Listen to your voice memos!") Or, surprise him by preparing a special meal to share and follow it with a dessert you can spoon-feed one another. If anything, you could ask him, "Babe, what can I do to make your day better?" These gestures aren't rocket science, just a little loving thoughtfulness that shows him he's still number one.

Try this: Do something out of the ordinary once a week that will make your spouse feel your love. I promise it'll come back to you in return. And if it doesn't, remember to use a W-word and simply ASK for a gesture that would delight you.

4. Create a Morning Ritual Together

A morning ritual can be as simple as rolling over for a sweet, sleepy hug that ends in six kisses, or asking each other the same questions before you shower. *Did you dream? What are you grateful for? What do you want to accomplish today?* You could even share a few things you love about each other. It might be that you brew his coffee just how he likes it and he makes your toast just right. Maybe you create a custom handshake that ends with a silly chant and a lingering kiss that you perform before you race out of the door. I'm fond of retelling stories of our best dates in the morning, and I'll often do it in front of the kids. I want them to see, firsthand, that our romance is alive and kicking. As mornings in a household with kids are usually chaotic and crazy, a ritual that's special to just the two of you will create a palpable tenderness and subtle flirtation that lingers throughout the day.

Try this: If you've already got a morning ritual, give it a special moniker so that it's unique to you and your spouse. Having something that connects you will unite you as a team each and every morning, warming your hearts (and reigniting your Mojo!) as the years go by.

5. Show Up and Show Support

Simply *show up and watch your spouse do what he does best.* You do it for the kids, *all the time,* so why not for your man? For example, if your partner is really good at tennis, surprise him and turn up to a match or lesson. Make eye contact and show him that you're impressed and turned on by his athletic abilities. Showing up shows him you think he's a hot, powerful, and talented guy, which gives him an ego boost and makes him feel like *the man,* which in turn, makes you feel like *his woman.* It's so basic, yet so effective in giving your love connection a boost. It generates butterflies, instant flirtation. You don't even need to stay for too long: even five minutes can give your partner the ego boost he needs. Bonus: You can take this kind of supportive flirting to the next level by taking part in the activity. In doing so, you're saying, *I'm interested in what you're interested in,* or at least you're attempting to be. And who doesn't want their partner to share their interests?

Try this: Show up to watch your spouse do something he excels at: a sport, a work presentation, even a hobby like building something in the garage. Throw a compliment his way and let him know his talent inspires you. Invite him to reciprocate and show up for something you're doing, too!

6. PUT DOWN YOUR F*%$% PHONE!

For heaven's sake, please stop staring at your screen and talk to your spouse. If you pick up your phone the first thing in the morning, break that habit and try cuddling for a few minutes instead. Or even read or watch the news *together.* If he's driving, put your phone away and actually talk to each other. Leave it to charge while you're watching your favorite show and discuss the plot twists instead of scrolling through your phone while you're sort of half-watching. Take away the distraction of your smartphone and tune in to each other instead.

Try this: Make it a rule between the two of you to put your phones away, even if it's just for one set hour in the day. Putting it away creates space to interact without distraction, and room for real flirtation to blossom.

But . . . will it work? Yes!

Remember, you may be parents now, but you were lovers first. Bring back that lovin' feelin' by trying a few of the positive actions listed above. Or, create a few that are unique to your relationship. Before you know it, you and your spouse will start to remember yourselves as a COUPLE, and not just as a parenting team. When you start reconnecting outside the bedroom each and every day, you have the opportunity to fall in love with each other all over again, again and again. You'll feel nurtured and cared for—and excited that you're making him feel the same way.

Don't forget that intentional romance and connection *outside* of the bedroom is a critical prelude to satisfying sex. It's the foreplay to your foreplay! Talk about your desire to choose romance over routine, flirtation over the familiar, and make an effort to do little things for and with one another each and every day—things that make you feel more like a couple, and less like two parents captaining a ship with little pirates running amok.

The Blowjob
A Sexy Session

I T WAS EIGHT-THIRTY on a Tuesday night. We'd just gotten the kids in bed and were standing in the kitchen, flirting and chatting. My husband poured me a glass of wine and said, "What do you want for dinner?" I paused, took a sip, smiled seductively, and said, "Your cock."

He let out a surprised laugh and said, "I thought you were going to say spaghetti."

It had been about five days since we'd last had sex and I could tell he was feeling frisky. However, I had my period, and while I don't usually go completely out-of-commission during my cycle, this period had been particularly painful with cramps and a nagging migraine. But that night, I was feeling amorous, affectionate, and ultra-appreciative of my loving husband—and I wanted to show it.

I took his hand, led him to the bedroom, stepped out of my yoga pants to show some skin, and pleasured him with a sensual blowjob. I teased him, touched him, and rhythmically played with the family jewels. But most of all, I enjoyed myself and made sure he felt my enthusiasm.

The act of *giving* took my mind off my migraine, and the raw sensuality and clear satisfaction of his experience warmed my body and relaxed my cramps. It only took ten minutes to honor his sexual desire and appetite without putting any expectations on mine. I got to show off my sexual prowess and received a confidence boost in return. And then, he cooked me an amazing spaghetti dinner. Talk about a win-win!

Let the record show that one of my favorite gifts to give my husband is an impromptu blowjob. Because blowjobs are easy! They're pretty tidy. They're quicker than a Long Love Session. As a mom in one of my workshops so eloquently put it, "I'm not always interested in sex with my husband, but I love to give him blowjobs. I throw them out like I'm serving pancakes. Here's a chocolate chip one in the shower, here's one with syrup in bed, here's one with blueberries on the couch. I cook, you clean up. I'm happy to serve you, even if I'm not hungry myself."

Blowjobs can be used as a tool to satisfy your partner's desires, especially if your sex drives are mismatched. If you love your man and have a strong relationship, you probably want him to feel satisfied, even if you're not interested in being satisfied yourself. So, *serve him up a pancake . . .* because men enjoy them—very, *very* much. Every. Single. Time.

Sexy Session #4: The Blowjob

Another important Sexy Session in this book is the spontaneous blowjob. This Session is a self-initiated treat from you to him, and ideally, it should happen once a week (your turn to receive is coming in an upcoming Session). It might sound antiquated, but I truly believe that every good man deserves good lip service as a delightful offering from the person who loves him.

Before you freak out and start shouting at me about *something else you have to do for someone else!,* consider this:

It's About Giving (Selflessly)

Men love blowjobs, and I LOVE to please my guy. He's a fantastic husband and father, and I like to show my appreciation for him in a way that's physically tangible. Because let's face it, in countless instances each and every day, he *doesn't* come first anymore. The kids do—and they often get my energy and attention before he does. But when I'm worshiping my husband's manhood, I'm essentially worshiping him *as a man*. I'm making it clear that his manhood (both literally and figuratively) is important to me and worthy of my attention. In that moment, in that offering, I'm putting him front and center. Because really, who *doesn't* need that? I'm nurturing him in a way he needs to be nurtured. And by celebrating and nourishing his masculinity in this way, it only inspires him to want to support, adore, and care for me more.

It's About Your Confidence

While it's no secret that a blowjob makes a man feel powerful . . . the truth is that it can be a very powerful, satisfying experience for you as well. When you give oral, *you* are in control of his pleasure. *You* are in charge of his most precious, delicate parts. *You* can practice and show off your Sexual Superpowers (more on that later in the book). You are taking charge of an exciting sexual experience, and because of it, your own sexual confidence receives a boost. I want you to own your power in this experience: it's just as much a gift to yourself as it is to your partner.

It's About Connection

The blowjob inspires trust and communication—both spoken and unspoken—between partners. It requires dedication, skill, and focus. It's a demonstration of love and affection and is a sexual act that says, *You're important to me.* All of this builds increased intimacy between you. This Sexy Session can be an incredibly satisfying and connected moment for you *together*. The blowjob strengthens your bond, intensifies your sexual connection, and increases your active participation in your sex life.

It's time to get on the BJ bandwagon! If you've fallen off in recent years, or never bothered to get on in the first place, now is your moment. But first, let's address some basic concerns that many women have to ensure you have the best possible experience:

♥ If he needs grooming, let him know or groom him yourself.

♥ If you don't like the taste of oral sex, try some flavored lubricant.

♥ If you're concerned about gagging, don't worry—you can use your hand and control how much you take into your mouth.

♥ Remember: YOU are in charge. Despite what a lot of porn tries to tell us—unless you're deliberately playing the role of submissive—*you* set the pace, *you* control his pleasure, *you* have a chance to show off your sexual prowess.

YOUR MISSION: GIVE HIM A BLOWJOB, *TODAY*

Today, your Sexy Session mission is simple: gift your man with a blowjob. Make it spontaneous, and lustily pull him away from whatever he's doing to the location of your choice. Or, plan it in advance: tell him before he leaves for work and let his excitement and anticipation for it build all day long.

Here is some inspiration to make your oral offering a huge and happy success:

. . . .

**Forget the fancy fellatio tricks,
it's all about your ENTHUSIASM.**

. . . .

1. THE ONLY TECHNIQUE YOU NEED TO KNOW

The key to any great blowjob is ENTHUSIASM. That means you don't have to go fast or deep-throat, or use any fancy tricks that porn stars do (although you can if you'd like). You just need to be fully present and genuinely desiring of the experience. He wants and needs to *feel* that you are passionately devoting your talents to making his manhood very happy—and that you're not just doing it because you feel like you have to. Because let's face it: obligation is a boner killer. No one wants to feel as if their pleasure is your chore.

Your enthusiasm begins with your initiation. Don't say, "Um, so, do you want a blowjob?" Practice self-assurance and flat out tell him, "I really want to give you a blowjob," as you start unbuttoning his pants. Or, you could go a step further and straddle him while he's sitting on the couch, pressing your breasts against his face, and saying something along the lines of, "I'm dying to taste you. I want you in my mouth. Right. Now." This approach will incite instant excitation in him—and you haven't even touched him yet.

Continue your mission with eager enthusiasm. Make eye contact that conveys your desire for him. Explore his body with your hands, slowly caressing his inner thighs first, dancing around his shaft, until you finally begin stroking him. Once you've built up tension, and he's standing at full attention, bring your mouth and tongue in to taste him. Release a little moan of pleasure when you do, to show him just how good he tastes to you. Continue combining mouth and hand strokes until you find the rhythm that brings him to the brink—but not to the finish line just yet.

You want him to enjoy the whole process—this is a treat for him, so give the experience some time to get interesting. Play with his levels of arousal: stopping, starting, then stopping and starting again, "edging" him in this way will make for a bigger, better, and more powerful orgasm. Pause for a moment to lift your body and come up for air, tossing your hair, touching your breasts, writhing your body in slow, seductive circles, and then whispering something sexy like, "You taste so good, I want more!" Then start again, moaning and lapping him up. Give *the twins* some attention too, lightly tickling them in circles with your tongue, or repeating a tiny upstroke like a cat lapping up milk. Never underestimate how good it feels to a man to have his jewels licked during a BJ. Once you sense he's getting close to climax, don't let the pressure of your hand and mouth let up, but boldly move forward until you bring him to a rousing finish.

Once he comes, *stay together* for a moment. If possible, place a towel on your nightstand before you get started, so you don't need to jump out of bed immediately to wash up. Trace your fingers up and down his legs and chest, and ask confident questions about the experience. (For example, "Did you like it when I licked you like that?") Use his afterglow time as a moment to cuddle and connect to strengthen your bond.

This Sexy Session isn't full of complicated tips or elaborate maneuvers—just genuine, generous enthusiasm. When you approach this gift-giving act of oral sex in this way, you don't need any fancy tricks.

(However, in case you feel you need a little extra inspiration to get you started, head over to www.DanaBMyers.com/resources for more tips and tricks to offer mind-blowing BJs.)

But before you go on a research mission, remember, you can always just ASK YOUR MAN to tell you what he likes, in detail, as you go. You might also consider watching some blowjob porn together. Ask him which style or technique turns him on, and make a mental note. Don't worry about mimicking exactly what you see onscreen, just take inspiration from the overall style, and make the maneuvers your own.

What to Know Before You Blow

♥ If you're really angry at your husband right now, save this Sexy Session for another time. Blowjobs and resentment don't go well together. Wait until you resolve the issue and reconnect emotionally before you try this Sexy Session.

♥ If you just *hate* blowjobs and cannot change your mind about them, make it an incredible hand job instead. Engage with the same enthusiasm described above, and have some lube on hand.

♥ If you're wondering why on earth you're focusing on his pleasure before yours, don't worry. Your opportunity to receive is coming. Most moms are more comfortable giving *first* . . . but as their Mojo begins to return by implementing the tools throughout this book, they become more ready to receive pleasure. If you're ready for it NOW, then by all means, ASK!

Remember, the Sexy Sessions are about reintroducing frequency, variety, and connectedness back to your sex life, and the blowjob is part of that. Focus on being bold enough to shake things up, to change old patterns and redefine your sex life—you've got this!

O-NOTES: KEEP A SEXY SESSIONS JOURNAL

It's time for more O-Notes. Once you've initiated your enthusiastic blowjob experience, jot down where and when you did it, what your invitation sounded like, how your enthusiasm showed up, and any other thoughts you had about the experience.

Write down a quick journal entry about the Blowjob:

_____

_____

_____

_____

_____

_____

_____

_____

_____

_____

_____

* * * * * * * * * * * *

Congratulations, Mama! You've cultivated a current of energetic sensuality in your body *and* in your bedroom, and learned how to talk about sex in a positive and productive way. Coming up next, you'll rediscover how to carve out more time for yourself with sexy self-care rituals, and practice receiving more help (and pleasure!) from your partner. Ready to take the deep dive and explore your Mojo so you can express your innermost sexual confidence? Then let's get to it!

* * * * * * * * * * * *

PART THREE

Explore Your Mojo

Create a Sexy Self-Care Strategy

ONE OF MY EARLIEST childhood memories is watching my mom bounce around the living room in a leotard and legwarmers, doing eighties-style aerobics with a girlfriend. To me, it looked like she was dancing and having fun—almost as though she were creating her own party. But what this dazzling display was really saying was this: *I matter. I'm taking care of myself. Watch and learn.*

And watch and learn I did. My mother taught me everything I know about self-care. She pampered herself, spent quiet time in solitude, and took pride in the way she dressed. She carved out space to create her art, she planned moms' nights out, and she often escaped for naps while my brother and I played together. She was available, attentive, caring, and engaged as a mother—but she also made it a priority to take care of herself as a *woman*, too. I was in total admiration of her—the way she emphasized self-care. It made her seem so brave, strong, and feminine. She put herself first, even if that meant she was temporarily unavailable to us. The recognition of her own importance emanated a self-confident radiance and a noticeably sexy glow. Her message was clear: taking care of your needs as a *woman* is the foundation for a strong, sensual, and satisfying experience as a *mother*.

When I became a mother myself, I followed her example. She was a hot and happy mama, and I wanted that, too. During my pregnancy, I felt hotter than ever before, and I did just what my mother would have: I exercised and ate right, nurtured my creative interests, took more time alone, got massages and plenty of rest. I'd have the baby and become a hot, happy mama—no problem! I'd find the time, no—*I'd make the time!*

Spoiler alert: It turned out to not be as easy as I thought it would be.

When I had our baby, there was suddenly a tiny human that needed something from me every single second of the day—*and night*. Not only did this leave very little time for self-care, but also very little energy to motivate myself to make any time for me at all.

More so, I genuinely wanted to pour every ounce of my being into the baby. It was a primal instinct to give so much of myself with such intensity. I didn't know I'd feel chest-crushing guilt for taking time away to care for myself, or that feeling so sleep-deprived could trick me into thinking I didn't *need* to. Confused and exhausted, I called my mom and asked her how I was supposed to take care of not only the baby and myself, but also my relationship and my sexy confidence as a woman all at the same time?

She said to me, "Put yourself first, in small ways, every single day. Wear lipstick in your bathrobe. Stretch while you're cooking. DIVE into bed whenever you see the opportunity for a nap. Wear something pretty, even if it's just to clean the house. Put them in front of *Sesame Street* and do your work! Everything—and everyone else's needs—will fall into place when you feel filled up, rested, and have given yourself some quality attention."

Okay, but if I have to put myself first, then what was that crazy baby tunnel vision instinct I was experiencing? Isn't a mother supposed to be selfless, all-giving, and utterly devoted to her children?

According to my mother, the answer is no.

There was no way I could keep up with the demands of motherhood and still be joyful and present if I didn't take care of myself first. I could forget about striking a balance between motherhood, career, and marriage if I didn't nourish my mind, body, and soul. And as a woman deeply committed to her sensuality and sex life, there was no way I could sustain a healthy libido if I left myself running on empty, serving everyone else but myself.

A tired and achy body doesn't crave sex. A depleted, disenchanted mama will eventually start to resent her relationship. But a woman who nurtures her inner spark and sense of self is a woman who brings bliss and pleasure into her experience of motherhood and marriage. She's a woman with vitality, sanity, and sensuality—who knows there's always enough time for *her*, because she's made it so.

. . . .

Self-care is not selfish.
It's an important act of self-love.

. . . .

Take Care of Yourself First

After that clarifying conversation with my mom, I committed to putting myself first for my own well-being and for that of my family. But I didn't wave a magic wand and create a self-care practice out of thin air—I got organized and mapped it out for myself.

I opened up a page in my journal and began sketching out what an ideal, sexy self-care practice would look like. I thought about the questions: How can I help myself feel sexy, sane, fit, free, and tuned into myself with the limited time that I have? What areas of self-care will have the biggest impact on me as a mom, woman, and wife? When can I create these opportunities in my week? How will I make them happen?

What emerged was, in essence, a laundry list of self-care opportunities to explore, to nourish and inspire me, and help me feel rested, relaxed, connected, beautiful, and, of course, sensually alive. This master list became a reference guide to sensual postpartum self-care. At the top of the page, I wrote, *If Mama's Not Happy, Nobody's Happy.*

As it turned out, writing these things down helped make them a very real part of my routine. With this list as my road map, and the discipline to act on it, I made Sexy Self-Care a habit within my day-to-day experience of motherhood and career. And you know what? It worked. No matter how edgy, irritated, or exhausted I am on any given day, a little hit of TLC transports me to an empowered, sensual, and appreciative state. Even today with two kids and an even busier workload, I still know what I'll be doing for me, each and every day.

Here's what my original list looked like:

I WILL NOURISH MYSELF

Eating too much junk makes me feel sluggish and unsexy. While I'll never deny myself sweet treats, I'll focus on filling up with healthy, nutrient-rich meals. I'll eat what my body tells me it needs—and try to avoid mindlessly stuffing my face with chocolate at eleven pm! When I nourish my body with the good stuff, I feel better about myself, amplifying the sexy vibes I put out there.

I WILL NAP IT OUT

I will make up for lost sleep at night with a daytime nap. Even if it's only twenty-five minutes of rest, a quick nap will recharge and reenergize the rest of my day. After a good nap, I'm much less frustrated with all the ToDos at hand. A little sleep refreshes my enthusiasm to tackle my work, and I'll have more energy to stay up and connect with my husband, too! A regular nap is my antidote to feeling like a depleted mama. (And whenever possible, I'll pleasure myself with a Solo Session before I fall asleep!)

I WILL PRACTICE YOGA

Twice a week, I will pass the baby over to someone (anyone!) and head to a yoga class. I know that sixty minutes of yoga is the greatest gift I can give myself because it helps reduce my stress, strengthen my intuition, and create space so that I can just be ME. Practicing yoga enhances my sensuality by connecting me deeply to my body. It's the perfect practice for getting my hot mama Mojo flowing!

I WILL SAY *NO*

I will say "No" to things that make me feel overstretched, be it kids' birthday parties or three-hour sales meetings at the office. (I'll send a gift in advance or make a call in over Skype instead.) If saying "yes" is going to make me feel anxious or unhappy, I'll politely decline. It's okay to cancel a commitment and care for myself instead! I'll feel less drained because of it, and have more energy for playtime with my husband.

I WILL GET DRESSED

The *look good, feel good* philosophy really means something to me, so I vow to only wear clothes that fit and flatter my figure—whether I'm up or down a few pounds. I promise to be loving and accepting to my body no matter what my size, and I will wear fabulous, flirty bralettes and knickers, even if I'm just in jeans and a tee at the grocery store. (Tip: A little lingerie in the daytime goes a long way.) Instead of stepping into sweatpants at night, I'll try to throw on a soft chemise and jersey robe, because why not feel comfy *and* sexy while we have takeout and watch a movie? I'll throw a splash of color on my lips to run errands or clean the house, because on the worst of days, there is always lipstick to lift me up!

I WILL HANG WITH MY LADIES

Connecting with my close friends and fellow mamas is sweet honey for my soul. I might even skip a nap for it. At least once a week, I'll plan an outing with my girls, even if it's just a coffee and we've got the babies in their strollers. My girls are my strength and my source of support! Hanging out with them means guaranteed, sidesplitting laughter and tears, too . . . which helps me release my pent-up stress and exhaustion.

Keep in mind my original list was never set in stone. Over the years, the list continued to grow and evolve to include more pampering, exercise, and even spiritual work. Now that both kids are in school, I have even more time and freedom to practice self-care! It's not a luxury to do this . . . it's a necessity. It's self-respect and a powerful form of self-love. And it's critical to maintaining my sanity and sexiness, keeping my cool, and staying connected to myself, my kids, and my husband.

THE TOOL:
CREATE A SEXY SELF-CARE STRATEGY

Yes, motherhood puts more on your plate than you ever thought possible, but a strong self-care practice is essential to maintaining well-being and reawakening your sensuality. It's impossible to feel sexy, free, and fabulous when you're working overtime to nurture everyone else in your life, but not caring for yourself. The good has to go *in* before it can go *out*.

It's time to investigate what sexy self-care means to you, Mama. This next exercise is about identifying and prioritizing the most important ways in which you can care for yourself.

Step 1: Shift Your Mind-Set

If you think that sensual self-care is only for special occasions, you'll spend your life feeling depleted, waiting around for that lone spa day to come and go. Forget that! Self-care with a sensual spin is now a daily habit you prioritize and commit to. On some days, self-care may look like an extra dash of rich, vanilla creamer in your coffee sipped in silence on your lunch break. It might be the extra sixty seconds you take to massage your legs, breasts, and belly with luscious vanilla-scented body oil after the shower. Other days could mean a sexy Buti yoga class and a fancy girls' lunch afterward, on a Saturday no less. The trick is to shift your mind-set to believe that you can make *some* kind of sexy self-care habit happen *every single day*.

Step 2: Lose the Guilt

If you feel guilty for taking a moment away from the kids to care for yourself, I have just one thing to ask you: *What would you tell your best friend if she said the same thing?* I imagine it'd be something like, "You DESERVE every ounce of self-care there is to be had—and more!" Make a conscious choice to speak to yourself in the same way that you'd speak with your dearest friend. Treat yourself with the same kindness you'd offer her. And just like that, drop the guilt! It's a wasted emotion anyway. Remember, if you're *there* for yourself, you can be more *there* for your kids.

Step 3: Make Your List

Sit down with your journal or computer and start a running list of self-care practices that make you feel amazing, sensual, rested, inspired—you name it. However you want to feel, list the corresponding self-care action that will help get you there. Describe what, when, and how you'll do it. Whose help do you need? A sitter? Your partner? Give serious thought as to what you can get off your plate, and to whom to delegate. Caveat: Your "how" may mean that dishes go unwashed or that laundry goes unfolded. Emails will go unanswered. That's all fine! Because the trade-off for you and for them will all be well worth it: a woman, wife, and mother whose head is clear, body is nourished, and heart is full of joy and excitement.

Step 4: Practice, Practice, *Practice*!

Each week when you sit down to sketch out your schedule, open your list and pencil in as many doses of self-care as possible. Keep revisiting your list and continue to add new ideas to it, until your self-care practice becomes second nature. Do whatever it takes to ensure you get a shot of self-love every single day! For example, head into work fifteen minutes late, ask a friend to do school pickup, order takeout instead of prepping dinner. Become a scheduling maven and put yourself first!

Notice if your commitment to self-care begins to fade during periods where your busy schedule gets even more hectic and give yourself a gentle nudge to get back on track. These are the moments when you need self-care the most. Go big and indulge in a full day of pampering with your girlfriends to kick-start your commitment, and then you'll be ready to get your butt back into gear!

Step 5: Share Your Self-Care Strategy with Another Mama

Call a mom friend and tell her about your new self-care strategy. Share the items on your list and invite her to make a list of her own! Ask her to hold you accountable for upholding the caring commitment you've made to yourself and offer to do the same for her. Sharing is an effective way to reinforce your self-love practice and help the other moms in your life to do the same.

Okay Mama, here's what I know to be true: *You are amazing.* Go on and say it, *I am amazing!*

So why wouldn't you deserve to be well taken care of? It all starts with how *you* take care of *yourself.*

The secret bonus of all this loving self-care? It creates colossal space for your Mojo to come out to play! Got that, babes? Now go on, take a little nap before you resume all of your mom duties.

Own Your Sexual Superpower

I GIVE AN AMAZING hand job. From start to finish, I'm in control and he's like putty in my hands."

"It's the way I voice my pleasure during sex without any inhibition. Because of it, he knows what to give me more of."

"I bend over and shake my booty in full view as he sits in a chair—as if he were getting a lap dance. He goes delirious, and gets a crazy lust in his eyes for me."

"I use my Kegel muscles to feel where he's at, to squeeze him, and to manipulate my pleasure—and his. It's like I'm communicating with my private parts."

"I do this slow, circular rocking motion while I'm riding him, which always brings me to a big, full orgasm. He thinks the full-frontal visual is the best thing since sliced bread."

"I invite him to watch me masturbate, and I go all-out in pleasing myself—I actually pretend he's not there. It's a voyeuristic experience that feels much naughtier than our routine sex, like a secret treat he gets to see."

Whoa.

No, these are not confessionals made by porn stars. Each and every one of those proclamations were made by moms, moms who've harnessed their Sexual Superpower.

What is a Sexual Superpower, you might ask?

A Sexual Superpower is the outward expression of your inner sexual confidence. It's that thing you do that drives your partner wild. It's the move known only to you and your partner that makes an appearance whenever you're fully embracing and embodying your unique sensuality in the present moment. It's your sexual strength; that sweet spot you hit where you erotically excel as a lover. It could be a "signature move," like how you squeeze him with your sex muscles just as he's about to come, but it doesn't *have* to be. It could be a lusty look you give that flashes your burning desire for him. Or, how you *always* make the effort to grab him and sneak off for a Quickie at Thanksgiving dinner. Your Sexual Superpower is your own personal erotic prowess.

Unleashing Your Sexual Superpower

My Sexual Superpower is my *enthusiasm*. It's my willingness to say YES to sexuality with an exclamation point! To say *yes* to wearing a crotchless fishnet body stocking at eight am on a Monday, just because the kids are back to school and we finally have some private time. To say *yes* to initiating sex within our marriage as equals, because the responsibility is on both of us. To experimenting with wild and weird toys. To prioritizing our sexual connection again and again—through all the dips and dives of a long-term relationship.

This is not to say that I've never said *no* to sex. Or that I've never experienced long dry spells that took a whole lot of effort to find my way back from. But at the end of the day, my governing philosophy is to say a hearty *yes*: to myself and my husband, to the adventure—to the healing, magic, and connection that sex brings into my life. And that *feels* like a Superpower, both to me and my husband, especially now that I'm a busy, working mom operating on six hours of sleep a night if I'm lucky. My husband loves my enthusiasm—that I've maintained *and* evolved my sexuality through childbirth and the relentless grind of parenthood.

Owning Your Sexual Superpower

Here's the thing: I believe that confidence is the sexiest thing a woman can have.

You've heard this before, but now is when the truth *really* starts to sink in. Standing up and owning your own Sexual Superpower can be a radical confidence booster. Focusing on where you shine in the bedroom can help you overcome sexual shyness. That inhibition that may have crept in since you had babies is holding you back from fully regaining and expressing your sensuality. But not anymore!

And here's another amazing bonus: taking pride in your Sexual Superpower can be a powerful libido booster. That's right. When you experience your power to give and receive pleasure in such a visceral way, you'll drop your inhibitions and want to do it more. Boosting your arousal is a multilayered process. Identifying and taking ownership of what's *already* great is an important part of it. And c'mon, we give ourselves credit for the lunches we pack, the birthday parties we throw, and the deals we land at work . . . it's high time to also give ourselves props for our sensual prowess and sexual magic!

. . . .

Rock your Sexual Superpower, Mama!
When you own your sexual prowess, you'll boost your
sexy self-confidence and reignite your libido!

. . . .

Harnessing Your Sexual Superpower

What I love about this sexy tool is that it's not about enhancing or improving yourself, scheduling in sex or changing your ways. It's simply about investigating, acknowledging, and owning something that *already exists within you*. Now, I can hear some of you whispering, *Oh, no. I don't have those powers anymore. I'm too tired to show off for him.* Or maybe, *I'm a mom now, it doesn't feel right to have wild, raunchy sex anymore.*

Even if you've never spoken it out loud or shared over coffee at baby group, I promise you . . . *Your Sexual Superpower already exists.* I'll prove it to you right now.

AN EXERCISE:
EXPLORE YOUR SEXUAL SUPERPOWER

It's time to identify and claim your Sexual Superpower using the worksheet below. I want you to own your sexuality. Wear it on your sleeve like an invisible secret badge only you know about. Let it put a sly smile on your face when you think of it as you walk down the street . . . and then enthusiastically unleash it on your partner this week like the superheroine you are.

Answer the questions to explore your signature sex move, enthusiastic maneuver, or sensual approach—the thing you do that drives your partner wild . . . and in return gives you a strong sense of sensual pride and confidence.

This exercise is about straight-up bragging about yourself *to* yourself. So don't hold back! This is not the time to be humble or play small.

If you are feeling shy about this exercise, imagine how you might channel that into your Superpower. *Own your awkwardness*: it may be part of your sensual charm. *Embrace your erotic self*: it's yours and no one else's. Whoever it is that you are, become more confident in your unique sexiness.

1. What is your Sexual Superpower? Explain in detail. A good way to do this is to just focus on whatever sexual act you enjoy the most. If you enjoy it, chances are you're very good at it! Reference the statements at the start of this tool for more inspiration.

_____

_____

_____

_____

2. How does your Sexual Superpower make your lover react? What does he say or do in the moment that lets you know how powerful it is?

_____

_____

_____

_____

3. How does it make you feel when you unleash your Sexual Superpower?

_____

_____

_____

_____

_____

4. Can't choose just one? List even more Superpowers.

_____

_____

_____

_____

_____

5. How do you feel when thinking about unleashing your Sexual Superpower(s)? What desires, memories, or emotions does it stir up?

_____

_____

_____

_____

_____

6. If you're feeling a little shy or inhibited about breaking out your Sexual Superpower, what might you do beforehand to bolster your confidence? For example, maybe you can give yourself five to ten minutes alone to do a sexy five-minute dance in the mirror, or you can skip ahead to your favorite steamy scene in a movie and let that fantasy take over.

_____

_____

_____

_____

_____

YOUR MISSION: Now comes the fun part! Lay your Sexual Superpower on your partner during your next Sexy Session. Take pride in the ecstasy you're offering and congratulate yourself for rocking his world. Harnessing your Sexual Superpower is major for your Mommy Mojo.

Then, share this tool and your experience with a member of your Mom Tribe. Sharing is a powerful way to reinforce the confidence and enthusiasm you gained, and help other moms in your life do the same.

Fantasy Fun
A Sexy Session

Y**OU KNOW THAT FEELING** you get after you do something adventurous—like skydiving or running a marathon, or *giving birth*? The rush of adrenaline; the tingle of exhilaration. Pushing your limits boosts your confidence and makes you feel like a proud warrior—like you can handle anything that life throws at you.

This is the same feeling you should have in your sex life. But after years of marriage with kids, sex becomes more routine than roller coaster, more familiar than fantastic.

If you've been practicing the Sexy Sessions in this book, you've already begun to reignite your sexuality and strengthen your intimate connection. Way to go! But, if you crave an erotic bond that's strong enough to hold you together forever, you've got to lift your lovemaking to the next level by adding in a healthy dose of imagination. **You've got to bring your sexual fantasies to life.**

Let's consider the story of Ruby, a Brooklyn mother of two with a fizzled-out sex life. After attending one of my workshops, she and her husband began incorporating fantasy play into their lovemaking routine. The results were pure magic; they experienced a wildly passionate sexual renaissance.

After twelve years of marriage, Ruby considered her sex life to be "generally stable." However, when I asked if she was willing to settle for "stable," Ruby admitted to a creeping sense of boredom and even angst about the long road of monogamy. She longed for an exotic and even dangerous connection—something fresh that would reinspire her libido and provoke a wave of new passion in the bedroom. So I pressed her further and asked about her sex life when she was single. As I suspected, her answer held the key to reignite the lust and vigor she was yearning for in her marriage.

In her twenties, Ruby traveled across Europe and voraciously sampled many "delicious man morsels" in the countries she visited. Because most of her lovers didn't speak English, sex was the language in which she expressed herself. "I got to love him and leave him, and then move on to the next country and the next lover. There was so much mystery with each one, it was impossible to not be turned on by it all," she told me.

Now in her forties, the days of raucous romps with strangers were over, but her desire to recreate that *feeling* remained. Both she and her husband were open to sharing each other's desires, and so she was honest about how much she enjoyed those hot escapades with her foreign flames from her single days. Her husband understood what was missing in their love life: the erotic and exotic—the thrill of mystery. Together, they were committed to bringing back excitement in the bedroom . . . but how exactly were they going to do it?

I suggested she brainstorm fantasy play, in an effort to create a sexual scenario that she and her husband could bring to life that would fulfill her need for variety and intrigue—without having to bring in a third person or experiment with an underground sex party.

In an instant, she had her idea . . .

Sex Session #4: Fantasy Fun

Over a glass of wine, Ruby told her husband her fantasy. She said, *I want you to pretend to be Antonio from Spain. I want you to speak only Spanish to me, and I'm going to pretend and totally believe that you're actually Antonio, my Spanish lover, and not you, my lovely husband, while we're having sex.*

Although he didn't know a lick of Spanish, her husband jumped at the opportunity to please his wife and enthusiastically rose to the occasion. He dressed differently, learned some seductive phrases for the encounter, and fully played along to bring her fantasy to life. She let her mind and body get carried away, and pretended he was a fresh, young lover. It took a bit of practice to "stay in character" for the whole Session, but eventually, it did the trick. Her enthusiasm for sex within a marriage was reinstated, and her frustration with monogamy faded away. Now, *Antonio* comes out to play once a month, with *Jean-Pierre* from Paris and *Giovanni* from Florence making regular guest appearances, too.

. . . .

Use your imagination and have some Fantasy Fun—
the secret to a sex life full of variety.

. . . .

Not everyone's personal fantasies may involve transforming your partner into an international lover. But if that's your thing, then more power to you! Now it's time for you to discover your own Fantasy Fun, one of the most exciting, provocative (and to some, challenging) Sexy Sessions in the Mommy Mojo Makeover.

Whether we admit it or not, each and every one of us has sexual fantasies. But to what extent do we allow ourselves to let them play out? Exploring a fantasy scenario together is a little bit like a bungee jump in the bedroom: exciting, thrilling, adrenaline-pumping. I have found that many mothers push their fantasies aside, rarely bringing them into play in their relationship. It's as if they struggle to integrate motherhood with their innately wild, sexual side. I'm here to give you permission to fully engage your innermost fantasies! It's a key part of encouraging the erotic woman within and embracing your Mommy Mojo.

A rich fantasy life will make your Solo Sessions extra hot and steamy. By allowing your thoughts to go absolutely anywhere, you add more layers to your sensual personality. In addition, having fantasies and learning how to share them with your partner will nourish your relationship, build intimacy, and raise the roof on the excitement level in your sex life. You'll feel more confident in your own sexiness, in your desires, and in knowing what you want.

A Fantasy Fun Session will leave you and your partner feeling brave and inspired afterward, since you've both tried something new and exciting together. Giving yourself permission to explore and play reignites your Mommy Mojo and fans the erotic flames of your sex life.

YOUR MISSION: BRING A FANTASY TO LIFE

Set aside one to two hours of sensual playtime with your partner this week to do something racy and risqué, naughty and bold. You'll work together to discover, discuss, and act upon your fantasies as a couple. This Sexy Session will take trust, intimacy, communication, and courage.

It requires a sense of willingness to bring a sense of adventure back into the bedroom, and perhaps a glass of wine (or two), too.

Here's how it works:

1. Explore Your Erotic Fantasies

Grab your partner and two sheets of paper. Tap into your erotic imagination and write down a minimum of three fantasy scenarios you're each interested in playing out. Your list might include ideas like:

♥ Engage in a role-play scenario (Foreign Lover/Traveler, Boss Mom/Male Escort, Doctor/Patient, Military Man/Girlfriend)
♥ Film a naughty video together
♥ Threesome, real or virtual
♥ Sex in a public place
♥ Light bondage play (silk wrist ties, blindfold, spanker)
♥ Explore sensual foods (think honey, whipped cream, or chocolate sauce kissed off skin)
♥ Put on a strip show for each other
♥ Dress up in fetish gear (i.e., crotchless latex bodysuit, harness with straps and chains)
♥ Explore anal sex play

2. Share, Compare . . . and Choose a Fantasy!

Swap papers with your partner and—with an open mind—read each other's fantasies. Your lists will give immediate insight into what each of you desire by way of sexual adventure. This alone could feel like foreplay. Together, see if any common ground already exists in your fantasies—those are the perfect ones to start playing with. If there's not an obvious match, simply talk through the list and discuss which fantasy scenarios you might consider exploring. Work together and communicate openly until you can choose a fantasy that turns you both on. Remember, everyone has a right to their own fantasies, and shouldn't be shamed or embarrassed by them. This is an amazing opportunity to learn something new about your partner, so try to stay focused on the scenarios you're both excited to try for this Sexy Session.

3. Discuss the Details

Take some time to hash out any desired details, conditions, or boundaries you'd like to place on the fantasy scenario you've decided to explore together. Share why you desire the fantasy, what images and feelings arise when you think about it. Provide specific details on how you'd like your partner to please you during the experience. Talk about what you're comfortable with—and what you're not open to. Remind one another of the importance of *listening without judgment* in order to keep open, erotic communication flowing. Don't interrupt each other! Ask questions and remember: these are just *fantasies*. Just because you fantasize about sex with a lion tamer doesn't mean you're going to go and run away with the circus!

Here are some examples of what sharing the details of your fantasy life might look like:

Role-play

Babe, I want to try role-playing so I can step away from my day-to-day role of mom and discover the sexier, spicier possibilities within me. I've been thinking about being a hospital nurse on call with you as my lead doctor—you'd have to perform a full examination of my body even though we might get interrupted by an emergency at any moment. Or maybe a schoolgirl with my professor—you could give me good grades on my skills or send me to detention with a spanking. Or, I'd even like to switch it up and play a more powerful role, where I'm a traveling businesswoman and you're my gigolo—I pay you to service me in any way I choose, and I give you explicit details of how I like to be kissed and touched and brought to orgasm. I like the idea of exploring different power roles, where you're in control, and then where I'm the boss. What parts of these ideas excite you the most?

Virtual Threesome

So, I've always wanted to be seduced by two people, whether it's two guys, another couple, or even two women. I feel excited thinking about all those arms, legs, and lips . . . and all that extra attention being directed at my pleasure. While I don't want to invite someone into our bedroom, I read that you can have a virtual threesome over the internet, through one of the paid "sex chat" websites. We can find someone who interests us both, and they could watch us play, undress for us and take our direction, prompt us on positions or fun things to try . . . or we could all just talk dirty to each other and then hang up when we're ready to really get into it. If you're interested, I'd definitely want to talk through and align our desires and boundaries. I think I'd feel nervous and excited to get started, and then a little devious and wicked that we did it!

One Night Stand with a Stranger

I want to pretend that we meet in a dark, sexy bar or on a train home from the city, and our eyes meet and we just know we're going to drop everything and go have crazy, passionate sex. We enter your "apartment" and have a stiff drink, then you turn on some music and we just completely GO AT IT. It's a night of wild, uninhibited, totally uncommitted, hungry sex with a stranger. I want to drop the kids at my mom's house, and actually do this thing—show up at a bar, pretend we don't know each other, and tumble into the house tearing our clothes off. Do you think we can pull it off?

4. Get Busy!

Head to the bedroom or another fantasy-appropriate location and get busy bringing your scenario to life! If your fantasy requires more time and effort to fulfill, make good use of the time you set aside. Go to the sex store to buy props and costumes, research websites together, talk about which restaurant has a private (and clean!) bathroom you could slip into for a Quickie during your upcoming night out with friends. Let it also be known that not every sexual fantasy you mutually agree upon has to be achieved. Sometimes, just the act of fantasizing together is thrilling enough in itself—and leads to a hot and heavy Quickie, or deeply passionate Long Love Session. Go with the flow!

So . . . how was it? As you did with your first Long Love Engagement, celebrate the fantasy sex you just had by telling each other what felt great/weird/wonderful/comfortable/awkward, and *why*.

Remember: maintain loving physical contact while you're doing so. Then, get your next fantasy Session on the calendar. Because your body and mind are freshly lit up with pleasure and newness, this should feel exciting. Revisit your fantasy lists and choose the one you'd both like to dive into for your next round.

A reminder! Remember to stay consistent with one (or two!) Solo Sessions each week -- they will enrich all the sexy experiences you're having.

YOUR SEXY SESSIONS JOURNAL: As with all your Sexy Sessions, it's time to reflect. Take a moment to recall your Fantasy Fun with your spouse and journal your thoughts; free-form or by answering these questions:

1. How did it feel to share your fantasy? Bold? Scary? Empowering?

_____

_____

_____

_____

2. Did you act out your fantasy exactly as you'd imagined? Or did it flow into something unexpected, something that surprised you?

_____

_____

_____

_____

3. Did this Sexy Session increase intimacy between you by sharing something that was previously "secret"? Did it make you laugh? Freak you out? Or help you overcome any fears of expressing yourself?

_____

_____

_____

_____

_____

_____

_____

4. Did this Session open up new possibilities for pleasure between you? New possibilities for a regular practice of exploring your sexual fantasies?

_____

_____

_____

_____

_____

_____

5. Did actively pursuing a fantasy boost your confidence? How?

_____

_____

_____

_____

_____

Embrace the Five-Minute Face

I T DOESN'T HAPPEN OFTEN, but sometimes when I wake up in the morning, I look like a troll. Or at least, *I feel like I look like a troll*. One who slept on her face, in a hole, in a tree. One who got woken up by her troll babies several times in the middle of the night. You might know this fashionable look as the "squished face with puffy, tired eyes, and a visible double chin wrinkle." But, thankfully, there is makeup. And with just a little makeup magic, my inner troll transforms from frightful to foxy in just five minutes.

I have always *loved* makeup. I love how it makes me look—but even more so, I love how it makes me *feel*. Like a million bucks; like a beautiful, confident, sexy, and put-together mama ready for anything. Makeup is my mood-lifter, especially when I've run myself into the ground and all I want to do is climb back into bed—it's my secret weapon that boosts my Mommy Mojo in an instant.

This confident connection to cosmetics has always felt true to me—and not in any way superficial. During my childhood, I watched my makeup artist mother work her magic on her clients. It didn't matter if they were traveling businesswomen or stay-at-home moms, the results were always the same. A little lip gloss made women shine. A streak of eyeliner brought out their inner tigress. Blush perked them up as if they'd just heard good news. And a compliment about their beauty always made them sit up taller and more noticeably proud. No matter how self-conscious or self-critical these women were when they sat in my mom's chair, each of them was happily transfixed by their own inner and outer beauty as they looked into the mirror once she was finished. There it was: feminine confidence and joy unveiled by a simple beauty ritual. I was officially hooked.

A Seductive Beauty Ritual

Makeup became part of my daily self-care regimen as a teenager and I've never looked back since. As I've evolved and grown over the years, my makeup routine has become what I call a Seductive Beauty Ritual: a combination of sexy self-love affirmations and empowering thoughts recited as I paint my face. This practice has effectively transformed a mundane makeup routine into something far more special: a soulful experience that's meaningful to my Mojo, my sensuality, confidence, and creativity.

My Seductive Beauty Ritual works like this: As I swipe on mascara before work, I gaze deeply into my eyes. I whisper to myself, *I am beautiful and seductive. I am on fire today.* In that moment, I'm able to see beyond the hot-mess-mom stress, exhaustion, and overwhelm. I see my true self: a capable, accomplished, flirtatious, and sensual woman who is full of love, motivation, and confidence. In that instant, I'm no longer in a rush to get to the office—I'm in a *Mojo moment.* Or, as I gloss my lips before school pickup, I daydream of a passionate make-out session, creating a quiver of desire and a mini rush of pleasure. This ritual sets me up to take on the afternoon with a knowing smile and a radiant glow. A Seductive Beauty Ritual is not just about putting on makeup, but harnessing the power of sensual self-care. It's an opportunity to anchor yourself in self-love with a sprinkling of authentic, inner sex appeal. It's a statement that says, *I own my beauty, and I have the power to turn up my Mommy Mojo—to feel sexier—in an instant.*

My philosophy on makeup is that it's a creative outlet to express and empower yourself, amplify your natural beauty, and rev up your sensuality. Perhaps what's most magical about this makeup ritual is that it makes my inner light shine brighter, so much so that even when I remove it, *the light is still there.* And as a mom, I've got a simple makeup routine that's super-quick to do and creates a look that is illuminated, rosy, dewy, and youthful—with just a hint of drama.

I know that as mothers we find that there's less time, energy, and even money to spend on primping and pampering. We no longer have thirty minutes to do our face and hair, but only a fast five. But the truth is that we *can* get it done. Because **when we take the time to feel good about ourselves, it helps us take better care of everyone else.** If we've got the time for laundry, emails, and grocery shopping, we can find five minutes to connect with ourselves in the mirror to amplify our natural beauty, feel more attractive, and activate our minds and thoughts toward a more turned-on state of being.

. . . .

Putting on makeup is not about *being hot.*
It's about *feeling hot.*

. . . .

And I know you want that. I can practically hear you saying, *Yes, I do!* as you're clutching this book on the toilet while hiding from your children. So okay, Mama, let's get going then.

YOUR SEDUCTIVE BEAUTY RITUAL:
THE FIVE-MINUTE FACE

Here is a five-step beauty routine to look and feel gorgeous and desirable, all while boosting your Mojo with self-assured, sensuous thoughts. It's a snappy seductive ritual that will leave you feeling radiant, beautiful, *and sexy* in no time.

Ask your spouse to watch the kids for five minutes. If you must pick up a crying baby, experience has shown me that all of the following steps can be done with one hand. And if the toddler refuses to leave your side, sit them down with a makeup brush and an old compact of powder or shadow to play with. It'll keep them busy and buy you a few minutes to connect with your gorgeous self.

Step 1: Tweezer Teaser

First things first! *Grab your tweezers and do a full face check.* Clean up your brows and pluck any other strays growing where they shouldn't. Many moms start sprouting unwanted hairs after we give birth (thanks, hormones). But you don't want to discover a giant chin hair in the car after you've left the house, right? Use a magnifying mirror at home to catch any wiry strays before you put on your makeup. And keep a set of tweezers in your purse too, just in case.

Step 2: Get Your Glow On

Apply a pea-sized dab of BB Cream, CC Cream, or tinted moisturizer all over your face to even out your skin tone and give you a healthy glow. Lighter than foundation, these creams will give you sheer coverage, sun protection, and a super-dewy, refreshed look. There are plenty of variations to choose from, whether you're breaking out from postpartum hormonal shifts or fighting premature wrinkles brought on by chronic sleep deprivation—or both.

Make it Seductive: As you touch your face, sensually caress all the little lines, freckles, and perceived imperfections that you see. Revel in the experiences that put them there—you're a wise, sexy woman who's earned her tiger stripes!

Step 3: Say Buh-Bye to those Under-Eyes

Use an under-eye concealer or all-over brightener to hide the telltale sign of a tired mama: your dark circles. With a shade that matches your skin—or just a hint lighter—pat the concealer from the inner to outer corners of your eyes. If that doesn't do the trick, add an extra dab right in the center of your under-eye area. Blend to make sure it doesn't appear cakey. Next, take a light reflective pen or other highlighter and apply it right on top of the cheekbones for greater definition, under your brows to open the eyes, and in your cupid's bow to make your lips appear fuller. These well-placed dashes of highlight can put a sexy spotlight on your best facial features and really let them shine.

Make it Seductive: As you perform this step, look into your eyes and tell yourself you won't be this tired forever. Top it off with: *Damn, I'm still shining bright for being this exhausted!*

Step 4: Get Flushed

The whole purpose of blush is to mimic the youthful flush that signals fertility and sexuality. Apply a dab of cream blush to the apples of your cheeks for a gorgeous, subtle flush. I recommend an ultra-creamy formula instead of a powder, since the non-matte finish will leave your skin looking dewy and fresh—the way it does after you've climaxed.

Make it Seductive: As you circle your cheeks with color, conjure up memories of your most mind-blowing orgasm, replaying every delicious detail.

Step 5: A Little Mascara Never Hurts

Curl your lashes and swipe mascara onto your top lid only for a clean daytime look. If you want more definition, use a freshly sharpened eye pencil to line your top lashline. Use short strokes to hug the liner close to your lashes, starting from the middle and moving outward. Smudge with your finger for a subtle smoky look, or extend the line out a bit more into a baby cat-eye. Alternately, keep your top lashline clean and punch in a pop of color (like teal or purple) to your lower waterline if you want to feel just a little bit dangerous.

Make it Seductive: Imagine yourself beckoning a lover from across the room with only your eyes. Tip: Don't limit this micro-fantasy to only your spouse; it could be *anyone*.

Step 6: Love Your Luscious Lips

Swipe on some lovely, luscious sheer gloss to your lips for a juicy, irresistible look. Or, apply a neutral matte for a subtler sophistication. Berry, pink, red, coral, peach, or nude . . . there are literally thousands of shades to explore and finishes to try like matte, sheer, gloss, or shimmer. Whatever you do, don't default to wearing the same lipstick you've had in your purse for the last six years.

Make it Seductive: As you apply, smile, pout, and purse your lips, open them slightly as if you're ready to be kissed. Take this moment to connect with the sensual organ that has the power to express your truth *and* receive loads of sensual pleasure. Take it one step further and recall the best kiss you ever had.

Step 7: Put on the Finishing Touches

After I do my face, I slather some lotion all over my body, paying extra attention to the wobbly bits I may have been criticizing just prior, and then dab on a bit of my favorite perfume. Then I'll usually snap a selfie because if I'm feeling like a hot mama, why not capture that moment to remind me on a day when I'm not feeling so hot. Lastly, I send that picture to another mom friend with a good morning shout-out and a compliment, like "Thinking of you, hot stuff, and what an amazing mama you are!" Remember that it's important to keep sharing those good vibes with your Mom Tribe!

Looking Good and Feeling Great

It's undeniable that true beauty comes from within, but we can't argue that when we look good, we feel pretty damn good too. Taking five minutes to put on makeup will go a long way toward energizing your day when you only got five hours of sleep (no more troll-face!). Taking the time to prepare yourself with a Seductive Beauty Ritual will enhance your sexual energy, too. You may not have time to shower. You might even put on the exact same outfit you wore yesterday. But when your face looks flawless and you've empowered yourself with some positive, sensual thoughts, you'll feel tuned in and turned on. Foxy, feminine, and ready to take on the day, you'll rock your responsibilities and embrace your own sensual confidence. Now how's *that* sound?

Make a Love List

B Y THE TIME WE reached the milestone of our son's first birthday, things were really good. We'd gotten the hang of this whole parenting thing. We were finally sleeping through the night and experiencing a blossoming sex life. By two years, wow, we were home free! We had a loving, trusting nanny who helped us with our boy, and a magnificent sense of freedom in our parenting routine. There was plenty of time to spend with the kid and on our own as a couple, not to mention what seemed like an abundance of time to cultivate our individual interests. We were officially out of the new parent fog and had hit a remarkably sweet spot.

And then, *poof*—just like that it was gone. We had another baby! Not only did we find ourselves back at square one, it was more like square one times two. Or three. Because having two kids was not quite the "double the fun" I'd envisioned—it was actually more like quadruple the work! Don't get me wrong, of course I fell madly, deeply, passionately in love with my baby girl, and I beamed with pride over our newly expanded family of four. I was in awe of how our son quickly took to being a big brother, sweet and gentle in the way he connected to her. The miracle of life, love, and family was so real and beautiful. There was so much we had gained with our newest addition!

But damn—the sleep deprivation alone was awful. The fresh waves of resentment and unmet needs came crashing back onto us. The unnecessary and often irrational blaming and scorekeeping reared its head in full force! There was a sudden loss of free time, me-time, we-time, plus added financial stress and communication breakdowns. We quickly went from a sweet spot to a not-so-hot spot in a matter of months.

Although we were bonding as a newly expanded family, the shift from one to two kids distracted us from our appreciation of one another, despite our affections. In the midst of constant negotiations with a toddler and around-the-clock care for a newborn, it was often easier to focus on the negatives than to find inspiration in the depth and richness of our love for each other.

Checking In: How Deep Is Your Love?

Thankfully, we knew the newborn phase would pass and that we would be able to adjust more quickly because we were no longer first-time parents. But we didn't just sit around and *wait* for that to happen. We decided we needed a Love Check-In: a sit-down exploration of why we fell in love in the first place and what had held us together thus far. We would define the foundation on which our successful and happy relationship was built. We knew this kind of in-depth, intimate chat would help reduce the resentment that had resurfaced since our daughter arrived and restore our bond during this particularly chaotic moment in our lives.

Over multiple glasses of wine and bowls of takeout noodles, we dug in and discussed our strong suits. Like detectives with a magnifying glass, we looked closely at the keys to our success as a couple. We were making a Love List of sorts, a living, breathing documentation that we could revisit and get inspired by whenever times got tough. Because in any long-term relationship, after the electricity and urgency has faded, we knew that our love could fuel lust; that sweetness underpins seduction; and that the strength of our devotion is what keeps our sex life so satisfying.

So we asked each other, *what do we appreciate most about our relationship? What anchors us, binds us, inspires us . . . to keep our love story going, year after year, kid after kid?*

Here's what we came up with:

LOVE CONQUERS ALL

LOVE is the force that keeps us together when everything else feels like it's becoming a holy mess. No matter what the issue, however big or small, we commit to getting through it together, with love (and respect!) as our guiding light because that's what matters to us the most. Our love is bigger and stronger than any grievance or challenge, and so in the face of a problem, we remember to ask ourselves, *how can we bring more love to this situation? How can love lead us out of our anger, frustration, or resentment?* When we return to love, everything feels easier in an instant.

HONEST COMMUNICATION

We believe that honest communication reigns supreme. There's simply no "cold shouldering" in our household, no allowing issues to loom between us; the success of our marriage depends on airing things out, as soon as they arise. It's simple: our openness in communication keeps a clear channel between us for more love to flow. Although the truth can sometimes feel scary to express, it always leads to a deepening of our relationship.

FREEDOM

As much as we love to be together, we also value our freedom and independence. We both have a need for deep intimacy and absolute liberty. This means we support each other's interests, hobbies, passions, and projects. We encourage each other to take solo trips, and we don't keep score as to who takes more. We don't believe in restricting each other, and don't require permission to do as we please. That said, we *always* consider the other person's feelings and discuss our intentions before making any concrete plans.

ACCEPTANCE

Daddy-style, Mommy-style . . . it's what makes us unique! We have come to fully accept each other, and all the blessings and faults we both bring to the table. We trade irritation for acceptance, oversensitivity for patience. Because accepting that his socks will be on the floor and that I will probably overreact is easier than trying to change each other. It's a kind of revelation. But if one of us needs a kick in the pants to meet a personal growth goal we set for ourselves, we each know that a swift and firm, but loving, nudge is in order. We have to hold each other accountable.

CHANGE KEEPS US FRESH AND EXCITED

We have made many bold life changes over the course of our marriage—both personally and professionally. Some change has been our choice, other times, uncontrollable circumstances have led the way. He has been elated with certain changes that I have been utterly dismayed with, and vice versa. Although it's not always easy, we are committed to *being in the change together,* always as a team. We view life as an adventure, and that means we value change as an opportunity to continue defining (and redefining!) what our happiness looks like. Through it all, we are courageous, curious and we stick together. Experiencing change and newness together keeps us fresh, interested, engaged, and exploratory.

Our Love List is long and always evolving, but I found this practice so effective that I began sharing it with women in my Mom Tribe and workshops. I've guided many other couples to put this tool into action, and it's really paid off.

Here are few more examples from the Love Lists of some other couples:

Nicole, Mom of 2
FAST FORGIVENESS

"The biggest thing we value as a couple is that we never stay mad at each other. We go from yelling and screaming and even saying horrible things to each other, to laughing and hugging it out. Even when we have serious arguments, we refuse to fall asleep angry. We're just committed to fighting fast and forgiving fast as a way of life. Even if we don't feel as though we were in the wrong, we still apologize; the other person got hurt, and that's enough of a reason to say sorry. Sex is also a powerful healing tool that helps us just get the argument over with! We just don't want to be angry with each other in the same house, huffing and puffing and trying to parent the kids together—to us, that's a horrible way to live."

Renee, Mom of 3

WE SUPPORT EACH OTHER'S PASSIONS

"It's amazing to have a partnership where we so fully support what the other wants to do. When I told my husband I wanted to leave social work and pursue painting, he said, *Go for it. Don't hesitate. We'll figure out the finances as we need to.* And that support is reciprocal. He wanted to move the family to Spain for a year for his work, and while I was a little bit overwhelmed at the prospect, I said, *Awesome. I want you to fulfill your every dream. Let's make a plan.*

Jess, Mom of 2

FINDING THE HUMOR IN THINGS

"No matter what, my husband and I always try to find the humor in things. We laugh together, we laugh at ourselves, we laugh at the chaos and mania of parenting. A few years ago, we were close to divorce, but we kept talking things out and somehow, we managed to keep our humor alive through it all. Ultimately, I think I realized, *if I can laugh with this guy while we're talking about such dark stuff, maybe we can laugh our way through anything life throws at us?* Our focus on finding the humor is a real connection point between us—a strong tie that somehow can't be broken."

. . . .

*Focus on what your love is rooted in
and it will continue to bloom over the seasons.*

. . . .

YOUR MISSION: MAKE A LOVE LIST

Reigniting your sexual chemistry is only part of the equation. Often-times we all need to remind ourselves as a couple of the appreciation we have for one another, for the life we've built together and all the ingredients that make up our strong foundation.

Your mission is simple: Work as a team with your partner to redis-cover and reaffirm what makes your unique love special and worth continuing to nurture as the years go by. Writing a transformative Love List will soften your hearts, reignite appreciation, renew your closeness, and ultimately, inspire desire.

Although there are no set rules to creating your Love List, you will need a minimum of thirty minutes with your partner for it. Encourage your-selves to be vulnerable and honest, and to listen without interrupting, judging, or jumping to any conclusions. This is a fun, loving, collaborative process! You can even get creative with a big piece of construction paper or poster board, and use colorful markers to sketch out the words and images that come to mind as you go through this process.

Here are the steps to get you started:

Step 1: Get Warmed Up

Spark your connection to each other by asking the following questions: Each one is designed to help you tap into the unique memories and experiences that make up your love story, while also getting the warm fuzzies going.

♥ What are your favorite things about your spouse?

♥ How have you changed and grown as a partner since you became parents?

♥ How has your partner inspired you to grow since you had children?

♥ What are the most unforgettable experiences you've had together?

♥ What are the most romantic gestures you've each made to the other over the years?

♥ What are the amazing destinations you'd like to visit, just the two of you?

_____

_____

_____

_____

_____

_____

_____

_____

_____

_____

_____

_____

_____

_____

_____

_____

_____

Step 2: Dig Deeper

Next, dig deep to identify the core pillars that strengthen your love. Think of at least three shared values that drove you to fall in love in the first place and eventually start a family -- and have also kept you moving forward on this epic, united journey of partnership and parenting. Look at the aforementioned examples if you need help with inspiration. Then, describe what they mean in your relationship and write down the details.

1. _____

_____

_____

_____

_____

2. _____

_____

_____

_____

_____

3. _____

_____

_____

_____

_____

Once you've finished your Love List, post it in a place where you can both see it, or transfer it into a shared file you can continue to add to as new thoughts come up. Then, repeat this check-in process once a month, or every few months, to continue acknowledging and appreciating your unique love for each other.

The experience of being vulnerable and communicating in a new way can be a little uncomfortable at first. But with practice it will become your new normal, and even carry a richness that you'll ultimately both crave sharing with each other. By tuning into each other in this way, you'll strengthen your relationship, revive your closeness, deepen your devotion, and embolden your commitment to fueling your love too. And from this place of empowered intimacy, you'll be all the more motivated to tackle those Sexy Sessions!

Receiving Pleasure
A Sexy Session

E VERY MONTH LIKE clockwork, I find myself in a real funk. I feel distracted, guilty, irrational, resentful, irritated, and totally, utterly creatively stalled. My Mojo is not only turned off, but it's completely blocked.

This isn't the kind of funk a manicure or meditation can fix.

So I'll usually turn on my Sexy Dance Break playlist with hopes of inspiration, and without fail, that's when something begins to stir. As my body starts moving to the music, I detect a hint of passion for myself—a knowing sensation of what is always accessible to me: my sensuality. A-ha! The light bulb goes off. I know just what I need.

I'll text my husband: *Babes, I'm in a funk today—my energy is BLOCKED. Epic Pussy Massage required ASAP. Tonight?*

His response is always immediate: *Your wish is my command.*

There is one night in particular that still stands out in my mind, when my husband heeded my distress call and fulfilled my need to receive pleasure. After we put the kids to bed, he poured me a glass of wine, put an open book of erotica in my hands, and told me to meet him in the bedroom in ten minutes. Slightly tipsy and already a hint turned on from what I was reading, I walked into a room full of flickering candles and sultry music on the stereo. Much to my delight, he proceeded to dance for my eyes only, pulling out all his best moves. He pressed me up against the wall and kissed my neck, slowly but with urgency, and began to caress my body. Then, he picked me up, wrapped my arms and legs around him, and lay me down on the bed.

He smoothed massage oil all over my body. He rubbed out all my knots, gently kneading every single part of me, *except* my sex. Only when I was completely relaxed, did he begin to worship my pussy with his hands and fingers . . . then, his mouth, my favorite vibrator, and also his manhood. (Full disclosure: when I ask for a "Pussy Massage," it means I want the full works!)

I was completely surrendered to receiving this sensual pleasure. By the time I climaxed, I was so relaxed and turned on, that I felt as if I were in some kind of sparkly, sexy, intimate trance.

Satisfaction was rippling throughout my body in blissful waves. Stress and tension had melted away, and I'm pretty sure I saw stars. It was as though the channel of energy from the top of my head all the way down through my core and deep into my pelvis had been opened and cleared, and was now beaming with light and energy. I burst out laughing, ecstatic to have experienced such pure joy, pleasure, and release.

Just as I had requested, this Sexy Session was *all about me*: my pleasure, my healing, my relaxation—my receiving.

. . . .

Relax. Receive. Release.
It's *your turn.*

. . . .

As mothers, it's in our nature to take care of everyone else before we tend to ourselves. We give and give, with compassion, offering everything we have to the ones we love most. Not because we have to, but because we truly *want* to, because motherhood is a blessing, a mission, a calling from the deepest part of our souls. But when we don't balance this immense maternal giving with *receiving*, we wind up depleted.

Ask yourself this: Do you ever decline help, or feel guilty when you accept it? Or, in the bedroom, do you ever feel as if you're not entitled to ask for what you need from your partner? Many women resist receiving this kind of epic sensual pleasure, or fail to ask for it in the first place!

By not allowing yourself to be the center of your partner's sexual attention, you're blocking your sensual energy, your flow, and most importantly, your Mojo. However, when you welcome and receive positive, one-sided sensual attention, you refuel your tanks, which in turn cultivates even more of your special mommy magic to give to others. Remember: A happy satisfied woman means a happier mom, home, and wife!

Sexy Session #6: Receiving Pleasure

That following morning, I woke up smiling. I felt happier, healthier, more grounded, clear and grateful, and even more connected to my loving partner. It was like my reset button had been pressed. My Mojo was back! By receiving pleasure, I'd cleared the block in my sexual energy and had unlocked myself to experience my feminine flow again. I could once again give with all my heart because I had allowed myself to receive with all my heart.

And now, Mama, it's your turn. It's time to make *your* pleasure the main event, the sole focus of this Sexy Session.

Of all the Sexy Sessions you'll try in this book, I'm certain that this is the most important one. Receiving Pleasure—without any expectation that you'll "return the favor"—is a radical act of self-love *and* romantic intimacy, and it's beautifully, magnificently healing.

In essence, you're making a statement that says:

♥ *I know that I deserve epic pleasure.*
♥ *I know and speak my desires.*
♥ *I trust in my spouse to deliver it, and in my body to surrender to it.*

YOUR MISSION: GET SOME

In this Sexy Session, you'll practice receiving sensual pleasure without any expectation that you have to give anything back in return. You are offering your spouse an opportunity to be in total service to you, which could very well mean an epic Session of oral sex. Or, maybe a long, heavenly "pussy massage." Or both! It could also mean a full-body rubdown with no expectation that sex will follow. It's totally up to you.

Prepare yourself to relax, receive, and release—and be sure to openly and honestly communicate along the way. You don't have to please anyone else but yourself. Not your spouse. Not your kids. Not your boss. No one. This is wonderfully, delightfully, sensually all about you.

Here is some inspiration to help you milk every ounce of pleasure possible from this very sensual Sexy Session:

1. Explore Your Resistance to Receive

Does any of this sound familiar?

♥ *I can't relax with him looking at me so closely.*

♥ *It takes me a while to orgasm, and I feel guilty he has to be "down there" for so long!*

♥ *He's clueless when it comes to oral sex, but I don't want to bruise his ego by telling him how I actually want it.*

While many women adore oral sex and sensual massage and need it to build their arousal, others shy away from this kind of undivided sexual attention. Instead of denying yourself the potential for pleasure, I invite you to explore your resistance. There may not be a quick fix to your feelings, but expressing your apprehension can help you start to open up to receiving the benefits of this experience.

Take a moment to ponder these questions and explore the potential solutions I've provided:

♥ Does the idea of your man getting up close and personal with your ladybits make you uncomfortable and anxious? *Could you accept that your natural scent and taste are actually an incredible turn-on for your partner?*

♥ Do you worry about taking too long to orgasm, or that giving specific feedback to your lover could be taken as criticism? *What if you knew your partner wanted to spend as much time pleasing you as possible? And that he would actually welcome your feedback—because he wants to be the best lover he can be for you?*

♥ Are you shutting down because you experience guilt or embarrassment about sex? Or do you carry shame from a sexual trauma that occurred years ago? *What if you were able to embrace and receive this kind of pleasure as sexual healing and transformation, as forgiveness for yourself and others?*

2. Prepping Your Pussy

In order to be pleasured during this Session with openness and confidence, you've first got to show your ladybits some love and acceptance, too. Here's how to put your pussy on a pedestal:

Hold up a mirror to yourself and take a good look at everything going on down there. What do you see? How does she look? Wrinkly? Bumpy? Groomed? Pretty? Put words to your feelings, but don't force yourself to be positive. Honesty is important in this exercise. You can also try sounding out some self-loving affirmations to counter any self-criticism you may have. For example: *My pussy feels so soft and alive. She is strong and touchable. She is a lovely shade of pink. She is fucking GORGEOUS!* Then, integrate *her* as a part of *you* and try again. For example: *I feel soft and alive. I am strong and touchable. I am a lovely shade of pink. I am fucking GORGEOUS!* Your pussy is not separate from you: it *is* you.

Next, get comfortable with what you call it. What word have you used your whole life long? Pussy? Vagina? Honeypot? Whatever name you've given it, ask yourself if you're truly comfortable with it, or whether it's time for an update? I feel most connected and empowered using the word *Pussy,* but also refer to my vagina as *my Goddess, my Sex,* or *my Source,* or during raunchier playtime, sometimes I like to say *my Cunt.* The main point here is that you want to *own* your vagina—to infuse yourself with a sense of pride for this magnificent source of life and the ecstatic sensual pleasure it can create.

Now it's time to pamper your pussy so that you can feel more accepting and comfortable with your spouse or partner all up in your business. Groom your ladybits with a trim or a shave, or get a wax if you prefer. Have a shower before this Session or keep gentle, unscented wipes on hand if it'll help you feel more self-assured while you're getting frisky. Dab a drop of organic coconut on your fingertips and moisturize your lips as a pre-sex ritual. Above all, remember that sexy is a *feeling*. Stop believing it's about how you look! You have nothing to hide or be ashamed of. Your pussy is a golden magnet of good vibes and magic. In truth, you don't need to worry about your hair, your smell, your color, your cycle. Your pussy is *beautiful*. Step into your sexual empowerment by loving yourself so much that any embarrassment, shame, or self-consciousness will simply melt away.

3. Choose Your Own Sensual Adventure

Let's get down to some business . . . *pleasure business*! Take a moment to think about what kind of sensual pleasure you'd like to receive:

Would you like sensuous prolonged oral sex on the bed, as you lay back on a lush sheepskin throw?

Or maybe a relaxing body rub with scented oil that ever-so-slowly transitions into an orgasmic pussy massage?

Or to use penetration as a tension-relieving internal massage, after he's read you chapters from your favorite book of erotica?

Maybe you fancy something a little wilder or sillier? You could ask him to dress up as a gladiator, feed you grapes, kiss every inch of your body, and then seek out your G-Spot with one hand while working your C-Spot simultaneously with the other.

If you're unsure of what you desire, allow your mind to wander through your most positive sexual experiences with your spouse or someone else. What moments turned you on the most and led to a breathtaking orgasm? Conjure that image, feeling, or even specific maneuver, and share that as your desire for a starting place. Note: You don't have to know all the details of how this Sexy Session will play out in order to begin, so don't ever let your uncertainty stop you!

Now, write down the kind of Sensual Pleasure you'd like to receive below. Brainstorm a few details of how the pleasure will play out for each. This could mean specific strokes or kisses you'd like to receive, positions you'd like to be in, or certain things you'd like for your partner to say to you.

How would I most like to receive pleasure? List three ideas, with specific details:

1. _____
   ♥ _____
   ♥ _____
   ♥ _____

2. _____
   ♥ _____
   ♥ _____
   ♥ _____

3. _____
   ♥ _____
   ♥ _____
   ♥ _____

4. Express Yourself

Next, tell your spouse what you desire from this experience. Nervous? Don't be. It's easier than you think. You can share the notes you just wrote, or say something like this:

> *"Babe, I'm excited about this Sexy Session, and here's what I want: I want you to massage my entire body with coconut oil, spending extra time on my neck and back. When I'm fully relaxed, I want to receive a long, slow pussy massage, with some oral seduction too. Starting with my inner thighs, I want you to use long strokes with your whole hand, all the way up and over my pelvis, arousing me slowly, before you start stroking my lips and C-spot..."*

You can make your request as simple or intricate as you like, but detailed communication *during* your Session is also the key to helping your lover deliver the satisfaction you deserve. Let him know it may take twenty, thirty, or forty minutes of consistent, whole-body caressing and pleasuring to bring you to an orgasm, so you don't have to worry about how long it takes you to finish. Ask that he doesn't rush you, and also, that he reminds you to stay in the moment if you begin to feel frustrated or distracted.

Need some inspiration? The internet is a great resource for that. Research oral sex and sensual massage techniques that pique your interests; there is plenty of material out there. Getting educated on sensual pleasure together can be an effective tool to discovering what really turns you on, while adding new techniques to your lover's skill set.

Tell your partner that you'd like to give feedback during the Session.

Ask that he doesn't receive it as judgment or criticism, but only as your desire to deepen your sexual communication.

Don't forget to discuss the notion of this Session being truly one-sided. This Session isn't designed to be a selfish act, but rather, an opportunity to take a break from giving to everyone else but yourself. It's important that you stay focused solely on yourself and attempt to fully relax and release into the experience.

Obviously, your partner will also become aroused by watching you unleash your sensuality. So as much as he'll be committed to your pleasure, his body may require a release at the end of your Session! Talk through your options, or don't talk at all and simply let your bodies take over. Though you may have had the intention for this Session to be all about you, you could also surprise yourself by your own raw desire to get him off. You could also suggest that he masturbates afterward while you watch.

And a final note: If you feel you're going to struggle communicating *any* of this, and it's going to stop you from moving forward with this Session, just hand him this chapter and tell him to read it!

5. Relax and Receive

Before the Session, invite your partner to create a sensuous environment. Change the sheets and tidy up the room, light some candles and cue up a sensual playlist, and then set out your favorite massage oils, lubricants, and sex toys.

As before any Sexy Session, spend time loving up your whole self and take a moment to stretch, dance, soak in a hot bath, or read some erotica before you get started. Many mamas I know have a glass of wine or a puff of a joint (if it's legal in their state) beforehand in order to unwind and begin settling into a more relaxed and erotic state of being.

As you begin to receive sensual pleasure, stay present and focus on the sensations you're feeling: the kisses and touches upon your belly, breasts, neck, thighs, etc. Ask yourself, *can I be unashamedly present in my body, breath, and pleasure for this whole experience?*

If your mind starts to wander or you feel self-conscious about your natural scent, don't take yourself out of the moment! Even if you get distracted or feel guilty for the one-sided nature of this pleasure, acknowledge your thoughts, but let them go. You can silently repeat a Mojo Mantra to help yourself refocus on the pleasure at hand. Something like this may work: *My body is beautiful and I am relaxed in this moment. I deserve to be sexually satisfied. I give myself permission to receive one-sided pleasure.*

Practice breathing deeply and fully, imagining sensual energy flowing into your pelvis as you welcome in more and more pleasurable sensations. The more you breathe, the more relaxed—and turned on—you'll begin to feel.

6. Communicate, Communicate, Communicate!

If you are receiving oral sex, offer specific feedback on what feels good: what rhythm and pressure, what part of his tongue you desire, whether you'd like more attention on your C-spot or lips. When he's hitting the right spot, be sure to convey your delight—you can simply ask him to just *stay right there.* If you started with oral, but want to try something else, just tell him! All he wants is to see you in bliss, so let him know what it's going to take to get you there.

Do the same when you're receiving manual pleasure: request that he uses more or fewer fingers, that he props up your rear end to intensify G-Spot arousal, that it's just the right moment to add in a vibrator, or that you're overstimulated and want to take a break.

Every woman is different. What kind of pleasure feels great to you is unique to you alone. Communicating with your spouse helps him to become more sensitive to your needs and better able to fulfill them. By trusting your feelings and being brave enough to express yourself, you're creating a safe space to build intimacy and trust.

If you're not comfortable being ultra-specific with your feedback, focus on short phrases in the moment like, "yes, more of that," or "slower, slower," and even "tease me right there." You could ask him to "try one more finger," or put "more pressure downward," or "tilt a little upward." This can feel less intimidating than giving him elaborate instructions in the heat of the moment. Also, use your body to communicate! Undulate your hips when his touch feels just right, use your hands and twirl his hair between your fingers, then press his head firmly into your pelvis when you want to intensify his kisses. You can always just guide your partner's hand to where you want to be touched. If a particular touch feels irritating, simply move his hand to another spot. If you want to deepen your emotional connection, guide his hand and place it on your heart or face.

Yes, I know this feels totally vulnerable. We are not trained to communicate like this. In fact, we are conditioned to *not* explicitly express what we want sexually, or how we feel during sex. This is where your boldness and bravery come in, and where your commitment to reclaiming your Mojo must outweigh your fear of expressing your sensual truth!

7. Ready, Set, O!

Once you've been kneaded and rubbed, kissed and adored, and pleasured to the brink, work with your partner to have a stunning, majestic, body-rocking, mind-clearing, heart-opening orgasm. Note: Know that you are fully empowered to be an active participant, and can touch yourself as you build toward climax.

As you orgasm, allow yourself to laugh with pleasure, scream in ecstasy, or perhaps burst into tears, knowing that you've tapped into your powerful source of femininity, and fully expressed the confident, erotic mama you truly are.

Take all the time you want to rest and bask in the afterglow of your epic O. Invite him to rest in between your legs after you come, offering feather-like strokes to your legs and belly. Really allow yourself to absorb all the sexual healing you just experienced.

For some mamas, relaxing after orgasm can feel a bit tricky at first, especially if you're used to flowing straight into bringing him to orgasm after you've come yourself. Test it out and see if you can fully relax and be still for at least two minutes. Then, if you're authentically inspired to treat your spouse to an orgasm, go for it. If you want to experience the Session as a one-sided event, try that too! That may mean he takes care of himself at that moment, or later in the evening. Alternately, you might offer him a BJ Sexy Session tomorrow morning.

8. Practice Makes Permanent

Learning to request and receive epic pleasure doesn't happen overnight. Fully relaxing into the experience is still something even I have to work on now and again! What's most important is giving yourself the freedom and permission to try this practice. It's one that can quickly transform resistance into receiving, cultivating your passion for life, love, sex, and creativity. The best part? Motherhood suddenly feels a whole lot easier after you've gotten some.

O-NOTES:
KEEP A SEXY SESSIONS JOURNAL

As with every Sexy Session, it's time to reflect. Take a moment to recall Receiving Pleasure and journal your thoughts:

1. Did you experience any resistance to this Session? What came up for you?

_____

_____

_____

2. How did your spouse react when you presented your request?

_____

_____

_____

3. Describe your Sexy Session in as much detail as you can provide.

_____

_____

_____

4. How did it feel to have so much focused sensual attention showered upon you? Were you able to stay present in the experience? If not, how did you bring yourself back into it?

_____

_____

_____

5. Did any negative feelings arise? If so, what were they?

_____

_____

_____

6. Describe your orgasm.

_____

_____

_____

7. For the next Session of this nature, what would you do differently or improve upon?

_____

_____

_____

Learn to Love Daddy Style

THERE'S NOTHING THAT MAKES me fall more deeply in love with my husband than watching him in action as a father to our children. Just as I became more of a woman through motherhood, he has become even more of a man by becoming a dad. His flavor of fatherhood is incredibly masculine, yet it's also tender and sensitive. It is primal to witness. And you know what? It's totally hot and it turns me on.

Yet as much as I love and adore my husband and his parenting skills, I've also become acutely aware of a particular irritation . . . something I like to call his Daddy Style. Don't let the playful connotation fool you: Daddy Style is the unique and often maddening way in which he does things as a father. Simply put, Daddy Style is doing things HIS way, not MINE.

Here are a couple examples:

♥ He gets the kids into bed an hour past bedtime, after seventeen books, four glasses of water, three trips to the bathroom, and two extra cookies, on a school night.

♥ He coaxes our picky eater out of a dinnertime tantrum by teaching her to throw her food in the air and catch it in her mouth.

♥ He encourages the kids to toss socks at each other, instead of into the hamper, because "it's fun!"

♥ He gives them a bath and floods the hallway and also forgets to wash the shampoo out of their hair.

♥ He whips up chocolate chip pancakes for breakfast and then gives the kids candy immediately afterward, the morning after we agreed to cut down on our family's sugar intake.

♥ He jumps in the pool with them the very instant their dinner is coming out of the oven, and then kicks off an epic wrestling session the moment I give a *five-minutes-to-bedtime* warning.

Now, here's the thing: none of these are life and death situations, nor are they directed as some sort of personal attack on me. They're examples of my husband being an awesome, playful dad—connecting with the kids while also giving me a break from them.

So why does Daddy Style irritate and annoy me to no end?

I think the reason is simple: I've always been a bit of a control freak, and that aspect of my personality only intensified once I became a mom. Controlling the way things were done provided me with a sense of order—but on the flipside, it meant that if things weren't done MY way, they were being done the WRONG way. As you could probably imagine, this created a rather unpleasant dynamic within our relationship.

I started noticing my issues with his Daddy Style back when our firstborn was still in diapers. A couple times a week, he'd offer to run me a bath and put the baby to bed. But instead of accepting the help and relaxing beneath the bubbles with a glass of wine, I sat there stewing over *how* he was doing bedtime, because his technique was different from my own. Was he following the exact steps I used to pacify our precious child? Did he remember to set up the stuffies just so? And what on earth was taking so long? My inner control freak couldn't relax and I'd pry myself from the bath and hover just outside the door to the nursery, huffing and puffing as I watched the clock. Worse, I'd then bust into the room, interrupting sweet father-son story time to hurry things along and fling criticism about what he was doing wrong. Sounds pretty crazy, right?

Not only was I ruining my own sensual free time and being a total nag to my husband, but I was also shortchanging our infant son from enjoying his special time with daddy.

My inability to relax and embrace my husband's unique Daddy Style created a negative pattern that was not only bad for our family—but for our sex life too. Because how could either one of us be turned on after I had just unleashed a barrage of harsh criticism? This episode marked a pivotal moment: if we had any chance of holding on to the sexy relationship we wanted to nurture, my rejection of his Daddy Style had to stop.

TAKE A CHILL PILL

My husband made this revelation pretty easy for me, since he became very vocal about my controlling behavior. On several occasions, he actually said, "Look, babes, this is DADDY STYLE! Get over it. My instincts are good. Different isn't wrong. Accept my help and let me parent my way!"

I had to chill the fuck out.

While my killer control grip didn't loosen overnight, his message did ring loud and clear. I wanted him to have the freedom to parent in his own individual way, just as I wanted that same freedom for myself. I knew that underneath my judgment I trusted his parenting instincts. More than that, I realized that if I continued to critique him, it would only demotivate him from wanting to offer his help that I relied on.

Over the years I've learned to accept, embrace—and even adore—his Daddy Style. Because why be frustrated when you could feel grateful instead? Why be critical when you could show your appreciation? Why complain when you could celebrate his strengths?

The truth about men is that, just like us, they crave approval and respect, and want to feel appreciated. When you tone down the criticism, you create room for romance and connection. When we show our affections and welcome their help without judgment, they become inspired to try harder and do more for us. Talk about a win-win!

. . . .

Just because Daddy does it differently doesn't mean it's wrong.

. . . .

In the interest of helping you learn to accept your partner's unique Daddy Style, here are my tried-and-true tips for reducing frustration and increasing acceptance of the fact that he's always going to do things a bit differently.

1. Ask for Help . . . Then Bite Your Tongue!

When you ask for help and daddy steps in, let out an excited "Woot! Daddy Style!"

This will make you laugh *and* call attention to the fact that you are about to receive the help you requested, but on *his* terms. Whenever you ask for help, remember that you can't have it both ways. You can't expect him to help you *and* have him do it exactly the way you want him to! For example, do not offer a thirty-one-point checklist on how he should bathe, play with, or feed them. Bite your tongue and let him get on with it.

Make a concerted effort to dial down your irritation, especially since you're working on improving your sex life. (Remember: Irritation is the opposite of attraction!) You're in control of how you feel and respond to his Daddy Style, so you may as well do yourself a favor and chill out. Instead of huffing, puffing, and muttering obscenities under your breath as you tidy up his aftermath, try repeating to yourself, "I love him, I love him, I love him" instead. It may feel silly at first, but it does wonders to soften your anger and redirect your focus toward the positive. In helping you, he freed up your time to Face-Time with your mom or Pop-Out to your local pub with a friend for a glass of wine.

2. Accept That Done Is Better Than Perfect

Although we tend to think that *mother knows best*, what we're really telling ourselves is that our way is better than his. But ultimately, it's better that the task at hand simply gets done, even if it isn't *perfect*. However, does accepting his definition of "done" mean that you have to embrace the mess he leaves behind or the fact that your kid is bouncing off the walls after his pre-bedtime wrestling match? Yes and no. You need to strike a balance so that you don't pick a fight, but also effectively communicate your frustration without discouraging his help. Remember the W-words when asking for help picking up the toys or mopping the floor. Bonus tip: If you find that you just can't resist the urge to correct him while he's doing his thing, then leave the room or the house entirely!

Surrendering to the idea that *done* is better than *perfect* can help you:

1. See that his actions are driven by love—not an attempt to annoy you. Remember, this is a way to feel closer to him and receive his love and commitment to you and your children.
2. Relax. When you're more relaxed, you create space in your body and mind to feel sensual.
3. Take something off your already full plate.

3. Celebrating Daddy Style Differences

You may be the one who anticipates your kids' ultra-specific snack requests, coifs their hair perfectly, and knows exactly what size *everything* to buy them, but what if his way could work just as well as yours—if not better? The truth is that daddy brings a different skill set that is equally important to the care and development of your children. Letting him "do it his way" without your control or critique can help your kids build their own emotional, physical, and communication skills. Children need to prepare themselves for interactions with all kinds of people and personalities in the world, and this "training" begins at home.

Daddy Style differences should be acknowledged and celebrated. For example: While you're cooking dinner *and* helping the kids with homework *and* catching up on work emails, daddy might dedicate his full attention to playing with them. This kind of undivided attention from him makes the kids feel special in a different way than you can. While you're worried they might get hurt jumping off the pier into the lake, daddy will encourage them to go for it, boosting their bravery and sense of adventure. His tendency to let them struggle with complicated homework for longer than you would might just be building the tenacity and problem-solving skills they'll need someday in the real world.

I encourage you to stop looking at parenting with rigidity and start to find the beauty and value in his method—and then celebrate it. Learn to embrace and even adapt to his Daddy Style. Compliment him, build him up, and say thank you—A LOT. You'll receive far more help and support when gratitude is put into play here (and, of course, ask that he acknowledge your Mommy Style in return, too!).

The bottom line is that as parents, you're building beautiful, capable children *together*—and you each bring strong instincts, strengths, and commitment to the table. Life's too short (and marriage is too long!) to obsess and fret over the small stuff. It's so much less burdensome to soften up, become more flexible, and embrace the fact that there's more than one way to get the job done. I can promise you that doing so will create room for romance and more togetherness with the man you fell in love with.

. . . .

Mama, I'm so proud of the work you've already done! You've committed
to nurturing yourself with more self-care, realizing it's the secret to
rebuilding authentic arousal. Together with your partner, you recon-
nected both in and out of the bedroom, infusing your relationship with
more love, acceptance, and, of course, sexual creativity. But it doesn't
stop there. Next, you'll learn to master your Mojo, with two exciting,
erotic experiences. What's more is you'll redefine what's possible for you
as a woman, while learning to "see the sexy" in your everyday life. Keep
up the magnificent Mojo work, you're doing great!

. . . .

PART FOUR

Master Your Mommy Mojo

· · · · · · · · · · ·

Stop Trying to Be Perfect

RAISE YOUR HAND IF you relate to this kind of morning: I wake up at the crack of dawn, hurry the little ones out the door to school and then sit with a cup of coffee amidst a pile of clothes to be laundered, crumbs to be swept and To Do lists to be tackled. Suddenly, I get this overwhelming feeling that I am just not enough. Not enough of a mom, wife, friend, sister, daughter, entrepreneur, or business partner. *Have I inspired, motivated, loved or listened enough? What more can I give? Am I too bossy, too selfish, too emotional? Do I complain or worry too much? How can I be more like Kate . . . who's kids eat dessert only once a week? How can I do it all it better, more precise, more perfect?*

Despite what I know in my heart to be true, that I am a great mom, these racing, self-doubting thoughts about my abilities as a mother still continue to creep up to this very day. More than likely, you've been there too.

It seems like no matter where we look, there are opinions about the right or wrong way to be a mother: in parenting books, blogs, social media mommy-to-mommy groups, at school drop-offs and playdates. As if giving birth wasn't already hard enough! We are told we're not supposed to let the baby cry it out or switch to formula too soon and that our home should be perfectly organized. We somehow convince ourselves that our bodies will just bounce back and that our post-partum sex lives will be easy and natural. Oh, and let's not forget about advancing in our careers while still making delicious homemade meals every night!

The scary thing is that for every "right way" presented by one expert, there are ten other alternative "right ways" to do it.

And because of this, there's always another voice challenging you to do it better—which makes motherhood a breeding ground for insecurities and unfair comparisons.

Ughhh. Self-doubt is just so un-sexy.

PERFECTION IS THE PROBLEM

You know it as well as I do, that trying to do everything perfectly stresses you out and makes you miserable. Seeking perfection—while simultaneously worrying about what others think—drains your enthusiasm, crushes your confidence, and diverts you from your well-deserved pleasure zone. This constant comparing makes you feel less than. And it's hard on your relationship, too. How many date nights have been ruined by endless banter on what other parents are doing better than you, and judging yourselves as a result? And if I had to guess, there's a good chance that it's you instigating the majority of those conversations, while your spouse practically begs you to just let it go and unwind—and enjoy a date night out away from the kids!

Seeking perfection in motherhood and comparing yourself with other mamas can only do one thing: stress you out and turn you off. Our goal here is to turn you back on. Sure, it's normal to want to be the best mom you can be and give your children everything they could possibly need, but it's time to give up on this quest for perfection. It's one of the most liberating, empowering, thrilling—and yes, sexy—actions you can take for yourself as a woman, mother and partner.

. . . .

The truth is . . .

WE ARE ALL AMAZING MOTHERS.

. . . .

YOUR MISSION: STOP FOCUSING ON PERFECTION

Here are some tried-and-true tips to abandon your quest for perfection and leave behind the self-doubt for good. Steering clear of the comparison trap will not only make you feel more confident as a mother, but you'll also learn to embrace your true self. Because being perfect isn't sexy. Being completely in control of everything isn't either. But being authentic is sexy. Lightening up is sexy. Being yourself is sexy.

1. Stop Comparing Yourself to Other Moms

Comparing yourself to other mamas is such a tempting trap to fall into. There you are, doing your mom-thing, feeling super confident and proud and then you spot . . . *her*. The mom who grew the green vegetables that she hand-pureed into the homemade snack bar her perfectly behaved child is nibbling on neatly while quietly reading— in two different languages. Her hair . . . her outfit . . . and damn, her nails, too; she looks so good. Her kid seems *so perfect!* Suddenly, all those self-assured, positive bold feelings you were having about yourself just a few moments ago have vaporized and you've found yourself comparing how your differences set you apart. The crazy thing is, you can bet that while you're comparing yourself to that "perfect" mom across the room, she's probably comparing herself to someone else, too!

The big problem with comparing yourself to other moms is that it diminishes your unique genius—your particular power and flair—as a mother. It shifts you from feeling confident to feeling like you're struggling. Do you *really* need more struggle in your life? No, Mama, no you do not. In these moments where you are seized by a sense of crippling comparison, take a deep breath and shift your focus back to you. Tell yourself: *I am enough, I do enough, right here, right now, today.*

Then, recognize something even more profound: that she is you and you are her. Be bold, walk over and strike up a conversation with that mom and connect. Ask her how her day is, ask her for her three favorite parenting tips—not because you want to be like her but because there is so much we can learn from each other's unique mothering styles. Be excited about the beautiful differences that exist from mom to mom. Ask what her struggles are, because trust me, she has them too and she wants to share! Find yourself in each other, and allow the comparison and jealousy to fade away, making room for real connection and even a potential new friendship. The bottom line here is this: do you, and do it like a badass. While you're at it, stop comparing your kids to other kids, too. Your kids are amazing! Don't spread that toxic garbage onto them, even if you're doing it subconsciously.

If those feelings of competition stem from obsessively trolling that "perfect mom" on Instagram and Pinterest, take a break from looking at her page, or even unfollow her for a while. Search for more relatable moms with a social media presence who celebrates her mistakes and finds humor within the pitfalls of parenting (a quick internet search for relatable parenting blogs will bring up thousands of options).

2. Forgive Yourself When You F*ck Up

We all set high expectations on ourselves to do our very best. But sometimes, we *don't* do our best and that's okay. We scream too loudly when it was only a mistake. We miss an emotional cry for help because we were rushing to get somewhere we deemed "more important." We let an F-bomb fly at the two-year-old because they wouldn't stop whining. We shared a secret that we had promised to keep. We failed to catch them when they fell and they wound up bloodied and bruised.

Okay, so you made a mistake! Not the first, and definitely not the last. Take a big step back and offer yourself a little more kindness, and a little less judgment. You are only human, and remember that everyone makes mistakes. If the situation calls for an apology to your kid, be quick to offer one. I can't tell you how many times I've said, *"Darling, I'm so sorry for shouting so loudly. I was feeling short-tempered and I lost it. That didn't call for such a big reaction! I love you."* Then, forgive yourself and drop the guilt—you haven't "messed them up" for life. Kids are remarkably resilient, and they actually don't expect you to be perfect. In fact, showing them that you're not perfect—but knowing how to offer a genuine apology and learn from your mistakes—is teaching them a valuable life skill.

Making mistakes is normal; beating yourself up should not be. Forgive yourself, again and again, and remember that tomorrow is a new day. There'll be new challenges to rise up to, and of course, new opportunities to make more mistakes and learn more about yourself in the process. You may as well get used to it! It's time to stop being so damn hard on yourself and start to become more gentle and forgiving of who you are.

3. Lean on Your Partner for Support

It's an excellent skill to be able to process your missteps and forgive yourself, but sometimes you need a little backup. Your partner is there to remind you that you're still an amazing mother, regardless of the mess you made. Chances are, he won't see your "faults" the same way you saw them and will be able to give you some perspective on the actual magnitude of the situation. What you may feel was a disaster, he may help you see as a minor blip, or even, a character-building episode for your kid. When you're obsessing over a perceived "epic mom fail," a helpful question to discuss together is this: *What's the very worst thing that could happen in this situation?* Talking through the worst possible outcome will usually show you that the situation is not as bad as you thought it might be. Then, discuss ideas how you could better handle the situation next time. Not only will you feel better about yourself, but you'll be inspired to be more connected and loving toward your partner, too. Hugs and kisses are encouraged!

4. Celebrate Your Accomplishments

Every single day, jot down the amazing things you did for your family. Everything from *I breastfed thirteen times* to *I hustled for a paycheck that helps pay the mortgage*. Write down all the hardships, challenges and problems you encountered and handled like a boss, too. Then, give yourself a pat on the back for doing it all, with love and commitment. Like a real big, warm bear hug. Tell yourself out loud and in specific detail, how amazing each achievement was—whether it was the dinner you made, the sale you closed at work, the orgasm you had in a Solo Session, that your shaved your legs, or that you stayed calm all twelve times you told the kids to stay in their beds. Hold your head up high and recognize your supermom powers for what they truly are. Cutting out the crap you tell yourself about not being good enough, and replacing it with compliments about what you accomplished will help you recognize just what an amazing mama you truly are.

5. Be More *You*

There is nothing your kids and partner want more than YOU. The real you—in all your unique, and perfectly imperfect ways. So if you are wild at heart, become more *wild* in your mothering. If you are easy-going, then embrace it without fearing judgment from others. If you are artsy, adventurous, funny, lazy, spontaneous, intuitive, bossy, indulgent—bring *more* of that truth into your every moment as a mother. If you like to break the rules, then do it. If you prefer order, then bring it. Whoever it is that you truly are, share more of *her* in your parenting style, without giving a care to who is watching. Be unapologetic about it, and don't second-guess yourself. Although this takes practice, owning your uniqueness feels like pure magic. It makes mothering so much easier and far less competitive. There is less inner conflict, stress and self-doubt, and way more happiness, confidence, peace and passion in your every day.

By acknowledging and owning your authenticity and awesomeness, you're giving yourself, your partner and your children an incredible gift. As this new "be more you" mind-set shifts you away from the stress associated with perfectionism, you'll experience a renewed sense of freedom and flow in life and in parenting that will radiate into your relationship. Because when you're not wasting your precious energy comparing yourself to others or obsessing about doing things perfectly, you create space to have more fun, to feel more alive and to delight in the perfectly imperfect experience of raising kids with the person you love!

Inspire Desire

T RY AS WE MIGHT, let's face it: sometimes it's just hard to get in
the mood.

The good news is that revving up your sexual engine can be as
simple as seeking out a quick dose of *erotic inspiration*.

Allow me to share an example: three months after my daughter
Indie was born, I planned a double date with some friends. Like most
moms, I was tired from night feedings, my body was still bloated and
achy, and I'm pretty sure one boob was much larger than the other.
I felt awkward in my own skin and my libido was feeling rather lazy.
But it didn't matter—I was determined to go out and have some
fun with my husband. I chose an outfit that evened out my lopsided
cleavage, made my hair ultra-big to boost my confidence, and applied
my makeup just right. I remember looking in the mirror and for the first
time since the baby was born, I thought to myself, *Hey, sexy. There you
are again.* I strode out of the house with a rediscovered sense of sexy
self-confidence.

Then at dinner that night, I let out an audible gasp when my celebrity crush sat down opposite me. Leather jacket, Ray Bans, character lines—he was totally, spectacularly gorgeous.

And then, the craziest thing happened: he started flirting with me.

From the minute he saw me, he was *into* me, *onto* me, *desiring* me—lopsided boobs and all. With what can only be described as complete disregard for my husband, who was sitting right next to me, this devastatingly handsome celebrity began to shamelessly flirt with me . . . and I flirted right back. He locked eyes with me; his steady gaze burning through me and straight down into my Sex. *Zing!* Even my husband knew that this was the actor I'd been lusting after every Sunday night as we watched him on our favorite HBO show. And while I was somewhat embarrassed to be engaged in this sensual stare down right in front of him, he actually gave me a nod of approval, as in, *Go ahead, babe! How can you not?* The exciting exchange continued until we got the check.

Although I desperately wanted to, I didn't meet that sexy beast of a man in the bathroom for a Quickie, because I *really, really* love my man and respect our marriage vows. I caught my breath. We took a taxi home.

And guess what happened next? Super-hot, tear-off-your-clothes, kiss-me-up-against-the-wall, throw-me-on-the-bed kind of sex with the husband I adore.

That brief-but-charged flirting episode gave me an electric shock of erotic inspiration. It was an innocent flirtation that lit up my libido for *months*!

* * * * * * * * * * * * *

**Rev up your sex engines
with essential erotic inspiration.**

* * * * * * * * * * * * *

FANNING THE FLAMES OF DESIRE

Given that sex is usually the last thing on our minds, it can be pretty hard for us moms to spring into seduction when we'd rather sit in our sweatpants. In long-term relationships, you're no longer under the spell of fresh love hormones—that "new love" chemistry has grown into something more deeply connected, but decidedly less horny.

And so, you have to work on revving up your sensual engine. If you've made it this far in this book, then your desire is already rising.

Building your desire means to channel that part of you that actually *longs* for your lover, *yearns* for erotic connection, and *craves* passionate sex. In order to do that, you've got to seek out sensual stimuli, incorporating even more erotic inspiration into your world—actively and passionately. It sounds challenging, but the best part about it is that it can happen with very little planning or preparation.

Let's get to it then, mamas. Here are some surefire ways to fan the flames of desire:

1. Get Some Aural Stimulation

Instead of Netflix, why not "erotica and chill" with your spouse or partner tonight? Sexy literature can stimulate your imagination and heighten your mutual desire. While you may never actually make it to the end of the story, you'll always *feel* seduced when he reads to you and empowered when you read to him.

Here are a few more reasons to give sexy storytelling a try:

♥ They're an *instant* turn-on, a powerful aphrodisiac that can help increase sexual desire on the spot.

♥ They're an escape from reality into fantasy . . . and exploring fantasy adds rich layers of suggestion to your relationship.

♥ Sexy stories give you new ideas to replicate in your own Sexy Sessions. Think of them as an encyclopedia of seductive ideas.

♥ When monogamy feels really boring, reading erotic fiction together is an outlet to explore scenarios and imaginary partners that turn you on, but in reality, are outside the boundaries of your marriage. This is the practice of *creative sensuality*, where you both have permission to let your minds go wherever they may.

TRY THIS: ENJOY EROTICA

Explore erotica as a couple by trying out some short stories. You can do this individually or together, but spend some time bookmarking the pages with passages that get you worked up. If you have more time on your hands to read—and find you have an affection for the genre— delve into longer erotic novels, or even classics like *Madame Bovary*, *Venus in Fur*, *Justine* by the Marquis de Sade, or *Fear of Flying* by Erica Jong. Then, hand your partner an erotic story (or your Kindle) and ask him to read to you in bed, or even at the dinner table with a glass of wine once the kids are down. Want to hear *someone else* read to you both? Download an erotic audio book! Listening to a steamy story can be part of your foreplay on a Long Love Session. Got it? Good. Crack a spine and let the sexy words fire up your desire. (To get started, check out my recommended Erotic Reading list at www.DanaBMyers.com/resources.)

2. Check Out a Sex Shop

Frolicking around a seductive sex shop with your partner can make you feel like kids in a candy store. The experience is equal parts titillation and education; and your mutual, erotic curiosity will most certainly be piqued at every turn. And guess what? Curiosity is *really sexy*. It reminds you that there's still newness you can experience together . . . that *something* might just surprise you! Cultivating elements of curiosity and surprise, novelty and the unknown, are essential. You'll remember that your sex life and relationship still have the potential to evolve into new terrain, all while stoking the embers of desire.

TRY THIS: INDULGE IN SEXY RETAIL THERAPY

Ditch the kids at Grandma's and head over to a sex shop. (Do some research in advance for a modern store with a couple-friendly reputation and high-quality selection.)

If it's your first time together in a sex shop or you're a newbie to toys you might be nervous at first. But remember, one of the components to a great sex life is education! So hold hands, breathe, giggle, kiss, and muster your courage to ask a sales associate to show you a selection of beginner's toys. Pick them up, turn them on, and see how they feel! As you take in all the colors, shapes, and sizes, take the time to wonder together . . . *What does THAT do? Where would we put that? How would that feel on my nipples, his inner thighs, against both our bodies as we move in rhythm together?* Think of browsing a shop in this way as the mental foreplay before the physical.

On the flipside, if you're already sex shop pros, venture into the racier sections and see what tickles your fancy. Consider G-Spot vibes, couples' rings, pleasure sleeves, A-Spot stimulators, glass wands, and kinkier play items, too. Heat up the conversation with talk about how you might use several of the items you see *simultaneously*. Browse the lingerie section for a fishnet bodysuit or a lacy teddy with garters for yourself, and a pair of ultra-sexy briefs for him; for extra erotic inspiration, take turns trying on seductive outfits in the dressing room and giving each other a sneak peek.

Note: Most men would be thrilled to watch their partner pleasured by a toy and will want to participate. However, others could find this intimidating, as if it were somehow replacing him, or doing a "job" he couldn't do. If this is the case, put him at ease by suggesting it as a way to expand your horizons together and enhance your sex life. You can start with a small, non-phallic fingertip vibe, or even a pleasure sleeve—a soft, pliable tube with a textured interior that slides up and down his entire shaft and adds sensation to your handiwork. Starting with a toy designed for his pleasure will open his eyes to the playful and nonthreatening experience of using toys together.

---

3. Watch Porn

For many women, porn is a tricky topic. You might unapologetically love it (Yes, it's really okay to love porn!), or you may be interested in watching it, but shy away out of fear that your partner will favor the unrealistic fantasy of porn over his reality with you. You might also be completely turned off by it, recoiling at the very utterance of the word. Yes, there is a lot of degrading, despicable porn out there, so there is total validity to feeling this way. But not all porn is bad! There's also porn that represents the kind of positive sexual attention, pleasure, and satisfaction that women do want and deserve (porn has come a long way!).

With a bit of research, you can discover a wellspring of beautifully filmed, feminist porn that empowers the performers who make it and the women who view it. This is porn where women are sexual collabora-tors with their on-screen partners, rather than conquests.

And for most mamas, that's *exactly* the kind of porn that can fire up your desire. It can create an urgent, exciting sexual tension between you and your spouse. It can serve as education, offering expert ideas on positions, maneuvers, and techniques to try (and discover new things you just might like!). It can fill your mind with hot, healthy fanta-sies or even play in the background while you make love, setting the mood and acting as a sensual reminder to keep your Session energized.

TRY THIS: EMBRACE PORN

Let go of any fears, judgments, or shameful thoughts that you may have about porn, and explore it as a potential source of immense erotic inspi-ration. To get started watching, search for films by the award-winning erotic film director, author, and mother Erika Lust, or peruse my recom-mended feminist porn viewing list at www.DanaBMyers.com/resources. Open yourself up to the pleasurable feelings that come over your body as you watch the hot, steamy sex unfold before your very eyes.

Explore, discuss, and see what kind of porn excites both of you. Take turns choosing the clips until you find something that's a united turn-on. Search for clips where the female performer shares an authentic enthusiasm for what she's doing: she's vocal about expressing her plea-sure during sex, she's proud of her body, she's present in the moment. See if there is inspiration in that for you.

Note: If you see something that repels you, *simply change the clip.* Tell your lover why you didn't like it, and if he did, then ask him what it was about it that he found so arousing. The more you communicate, the more you'll be able to share in the stimulation! Give yourself permission to free yourself from restriction, and allow the experience to bring out the wild, free, in-the-moment pleasure-seeker within.

4. Try Sex Tech

These days, there's an app for just about everything—including erotic inspiration. There are apps for private sexting with your partner like Between, apps for inspiring new positions like iKama-sutra, and apps to discover and share your fantasies like Kindu. Ulti-mately, these technologies are all about improving your relationship and keeping things sexy, so why not use your phone for something other than scrolling social media and itemizing your grocery list?

There's one app in particular that offers in-the-moment erotic inspiration for those moments where you've scheduled a Sexy Session, but your Mojo is nowhere to be found. It's called Pillow, and it's essen-tially a choose-your-adventure game, whereby you choose an audio episode to listen to while lying in bed next to your partner (e.g., Hot & Cold: Teasing Massage Temperature Play, or Blindfold Surrender: Let Yourself Be Taken). You simply follow along to the play-by-play audio with kissing, touching, changing positions, and more. Listening to another voice instruct you what to do can take the pressure off conjuring up sexual desire all on your own, as well as create a swell of arousal.

TRY THIS: USE TECHNOLOGY AS A TURN-ON

Whenever you're feeling like your libido is nowhere to be found, download an erotic app and invite your partner to join you. Send each other playful, suggestive texts, peruse and rank sex positions or fantasies you'd like to try, or pick a hot audio episode and follow along to their seductive suggestions. You'll feel your Mojo rising in no time!

5. Get Your Flirt On

Who says you can't flirt just because you're a mama? You may be happily coupled up, but you're not dead. So go flirt with someone—*appropriately*. It's important to know that you are still desirable, and it's human nature to want that. You should never suppress your primal urges to desire and be desired; it's okay to feel them, just be careful not to act on them! At its most basic level, flirting is about giving and getting positive energy, and it's a natural, healthy, and fun part of any sexy, self-confident lifestyle. Obviously, don't jump into bed with some stranger you flirted with at the grocery shop, but a little bit of light flirting will fuel your fire, boost your confidence, and reaffirm just how sexy you feel. Then, just as I did after my celebrity flirting episode, you can channel all that fresh desire and sexual energy into a Session with your partner. Point is, you can actively charge up your turn-on by harmlessly flirting with others!

TRY THIS: FLIRT!

Flirt with someone other than your partner: a sexy server at the restaurant you're at for a moms' night out, with your delivery guy, or with an acquaintance at a couples' dinner party that's fully aware you're happily married. If you feel shy, don't sweat it. Just focus on being yourself and having a connected conversation with someone other than your partner. If you're unsure how to get your flirt on, recall how you used to do it: did you twirl your hair or hold a seductive gaze? Arch your back, touch your neck as you spoke, or bite your lips? Tell jokes or make coy conversation? You may be a little out of practice, but trust in your Mojo and flirt away.

Encourage your partner to do the same, but before either of you start, openly discuss the idea of harmless flirting with them: explore what the benefits could be for your relationship and draw basic boundaries. Many couples say that having "permission to flirt" keeps them from feeling trapped, offers a sense of freedom and fun, and ultimately, makes them appreciate each other more.

Bonus Tip: Spend Time Apart to Rekindle the Spark

As important as it is for you to be *together* with your spouse or partner— seeking titillation at sex shops and instantaneous arousal through erotica—it's also as important to *be apart*. They say familiarity breeds contempt and absence makes the heart grow fonder . . . but I think it's more like familiarity kills your libido and absence ignites your sex drive.

Because we know our partners so well and we're so comfortable within our relationship routines, there is simply no more mystery to be had. And that just feels . . . so boring. Yet change is sensually stimulating, mystery is sexy, and missing one another is a total turn-on!

So, in whatever way that you can, instigate change in your relationship by spending a little time apart. It could be just for a night, or you might even take a solo trip away for a week. You could try sleeping in separate beds for two nights, in anticipation of a scheduled Sexy Session on the third. Or, you could even agree to avoid casually touching or kissing each other for several days to build up the excitement. You'll find that a bit of separation breaks up the mundane and gives you a chance to miss each other and even *crave* the other person's company and sensual touch. What greater erotic inspiration is there when you can't wait to run into the arms of your love after a moment apart?

Mama, you're doing great; your desire is building. Keep it up by trying as many of these ideas as possible, and plug yourself into a source of erotic inspiration whenever you need it!

Playing Together
A Sexy Session

I HAVE ALWAYS APPROACHED sex as my creative playground—a place for fun, the jungle gym where I let my inner wild child roam free. It's a zone where I don't feel judged or inhibited, and I am always up for just about anything. Over the years I learned that sex was like a self-discovery lab of sorts, where I get to test out what is pleasurable and empowering, or what might be too edgy and uncomfortable for my taste. Exploring my sexuality with such openness has allowed me to uncover so many sides of my personality: the wild and romantic, the vulnerable and bold, the leader and the follower, the creative and the traditional. While not every sexual encounter has been epic, my carefree and conscious approach toward sex has helped to color my perspective in my life outside the bedroom as well.

This playful attitude toward lovemaking has been the secret to maintaining a happy, healthy, exciting sex life and marriage. My husband and I value the *variety* this sex-as-play approach has to offer. We are constantly introducing new ideas into the bedroom—some ideas we try once, others we bring into regular rotation because they're just so damn good.

Yet, just like every other long-term couple, I'll admit that sometimes we fall into a sex rut, too. We get tired. We get lazy. We fall prey to the feeling that we've already "tried it all" and boring bedroom routine starts to settle in. And that's exactly when we go back to the drawing board and revisit the idea of play, because we know from experience that *play* is the antidote to bedroom boredom.

Let me share the story of my longtime friend Jessica, a mom of three, whom I introduced the idea of play to help revive her sex life. Over lunch, I shared the details of a rather silly and sensational Long Love Session I'd recently had with my husband. It was, perhaps, a bit TMI, and she looked at me in mild disbelief and said, "Wait, where do these ideas come from? Do you just sit around thinking of ways to spice up your sex life?"

"Why yes," I said, "Yes I do."

"Well, don't hold out on me," my friend exclaimed, "I want some of that, too!"

Jessica's story is quite common: she experiences a partnership filled with love, friendship, and affection - but also boredom in the bedroom since kids came into the picture. She said that while they both orgasm each time they have sex, they always get there the same way. *Every single time.* Satisfying, but habitual. It's not that they were inhibited or shy in the bedroom, they just had stagnated into a pattern, and neither knew how to step up to the plate with ideas or the leadership to change it. So I dug deeper and learned that both of them had a regular Solo practice, and would often share a few details about their Solo Sessions with one another as flirtatious banter. *A-ha!* A light bulb went off.

I said, "Would you be open to playing a game of 'If you show me yours, I'll show you mine?'"

Jessica seemed curious enough, so I suggested they try mutual masturbation—the act of pleasuring themselves in the same room. They'd watch each other have an erotic experience of a Solo Session without getting physically involved in their orgasmic journeys. Although neither of them had considered this before, they decided to go for it and give my idea of a little playtime a try.

During their pre-sex discussion, they agreed to masturbate as freely as possible, as if they were having a true Solo Session. They committed to making eye contact when it felt natural, to avoid giving any kind of instructions, and to let each other know when they were about to climax.

She was surprised at how having an audience lit up her "inner showgirl," and she found herself changing positions more often to expose more of her body and increase his visual delight. She felt confident, mischievous, and totally in control. From watching him pleasure himself from the corner of her eyes, she picked up a few new hand job techniques that she happily put into play in future Sessions. He was completely in awe of her—as he witnessed how empowered and erotic she became as she brought herself to orgasm. The bottom line: the experience was thrilling, even a bit taboo. But most importantly, it was creative, refreshing, and FUN!

This, my dear mamas, is the simple but courageous power of Playing Together.

Sexy Session #7: Playing Together

Sexual ruts are normal, but that doesn't make them okay. A healthy, happy, lifelong partnership depends on continuing to reinvent your romantic connection and reignite your sensual Mojo. But it doesn't *have* to be a serious or difficult process—it's possible to *play* your way out of the mundane.

The time has come, Mama, to infuse your sex life with a spark of innovation by Playing Together. This is your opportunity to experience a Sexy Session built on imagination and novelty. Playing Together is a departure from the routine sex you are all too familiar with and help you branch out. Get ready to play!

. . . .

The couple who plays together, stays together.

. . . .

YOUR MISSION: TRY SOMETHING NEW!

This week, your mission is to begin the process of transforming your sex life into a sexual playground, where fun and adventure reign supreme. Integrate playtime into a Quickie, Long Love Session, or even as part of a Fantasy experience. Remember: It doesn't always have to lead to penetration or even climax. If you're trying something new and having fun along the way, then you're doing it right.

A note before we get started: If you're wondering whether this Sexy Session is different from Fantasy Fun, it definitely is. Fantasy Fun was a deep dive into discovering and discussing your fantasies, which helped to strengthen your erotic communication skills. The exercise of Playing Together should therefore feel more spontaneous and less scripted. If you love what you try, stay with it; if it feels *meh*, then abandon ship and move on to something else.

Below are seven imaginative and sensual playtime scenarios to try with your partner.

1. Switch Locations . . . and Positions!

The easiest way to refresh routine sex is to switch up your positions and locations, which can make your home feel like a playground itself. For example, if Missionary Style in the bed is your go-to, try Reverse Cowgirl in the living room (Reverse Cowgirl is when you're on top but facing away from him). If Doggystyle up against your vanity is the usual, try Modified Missionary on the kitchen table (Modified Missionary has you on your back with your hips at the edge of the surface, legs resting over your partner's shoulders, while he stands to thrust). Bonus: You can make any position feel new and exciting simply by doing your Kegels. Squeeze him in rhythm as he thrusts, or ask him to stay steady when he hits the right spot and pulse your PC muscles to steadily build your pleasure.

Of course there are thousands of positions you can try, so maybe spend an evening together after the kids go to bed and search the internet for more inspiration.

2. Play a Sex Game

Who says playing games is just for kids? A Sexy Game Night makes the pleasure and memories you create together more fun, interesting, and naughty. The goal here is to bring in a sense of mischief, expand your horizons a bit, and enjoy yourselves! Try out a classic game like Strip Poker or Naked Twister, and up the frisk factor by playing in front of a mirror. Or, buy a pair of Sex Dice and take turns delivering the sexy and erogenous actions as you roll (sex dice apps are available on your smartphone's app store). If a no-props-necessary approach is more your style, create an updated version of the *Newlywed Game*. Begin by standing on opposite sides of the bedroom and then start asking your spouse questions about yourself (*What's my favorite dessert? What's my favorite position?*) or your relationship (*Where was our first kiss? What was the craziest thing that happened at our wedding?*). For every answer he gets correctly, he gets to take a step closer to you, while you take off a piece of clothing. If he gets it wrong he takes a step back, and you redress, bringing a playful, teasing nature into your exchange.

3. Bring Out the Toys

"Do you really *need* to use a sex toy?" is almost like asking, "Do you *need* lip gloss?" In both cases, the answer is no, you don't, but they both make you feel incredibly good, so why not use them? Sex toys are tools for fun and pleasure, and have the power to easily shake up your ordinary sex routine. Playing with toys gives you something tangible to experiment with together and can even help you get to know each other better. How? Because toys are props that incite questions and communication during sexy playtime, like: *Does that feel good on your thighs? What about your breasts? What if I use it this way?* A solo vibrator, like the Smart Wand from Lelo, is a good starter toy to use together, delivering all-over-body sensations with multiple speeds and rhythmic patterns. If a basic vibrator seems old hat, you can try out a couples' toy, like the WeVibe, a toy you wear during sex for simultaneous C-Spot and G-Spot stimulation—an experience in which he shares the sensations with you. Keep it simple or get wild with toys—there are endless possibilities here, so why not play freely?

4. Word Play

Talking dirty is an effective way to revitalize any lackluster lovemaking, but many women find they just *can't find the words* when it's time to deliver the dirty dialogue in the heat of the moment! Don't get stuck in your head. Instead, keep your dirty word play simple and easy, asking your spouse the question, *What's the dirtiest thing you can think of?* as you begin your Session. Openly receive his response without judgment and be prepared for him to ask you the same question in return! If your initial reaction is to go silent, take a deep breath, muster your courage, and know you're in a safe spot with your partner. Then, say whatever comes to mind without embarrassment. *Being taken by two men. Watching two women have sex. Eating a hot steak while you give me oral sex* (Yes, that steak one is a *real* example from a mom who did this exercise!). The conversation doesn't necessarily have to go any further—the admission of your honest, sexual desires can be all the dirty talk you need to electrify your Session with a renewed energy. If this kind of on-the-spot, erotic chatter feels too improvisational for your character, try placing a book of erotic short stories on your nightstand and take turns reading juicy excerpts to each other.

5. Play Dress Up

It's straight up fun to dress up in a costume for sex, and you can get a complete ensemble like a French maid, naughty nurse, or sexy genie for under thirty dollars. These alter egos can allow you to abandon your inhibitions and really cut loose. Costume play can be very freeing and funny—laughs are almost guaranteed before you find yourself really getting into the role, like a sexy schoolteacher, for instance. Ask your lover to play the pupil, and bring in a notebook to grade his "homework assignments." There are plenty of costumes that allow men to role-play, too. What would you want your guy to dress up as? You could even ask him to surprise you.

If costumes aren't your thing, opt for seductive lingerie instead. If you want something risqué, try a fishnet body stocking: it's visually exciting, and brings a sense of raunchy naughtiness to your playtime session. If you prefer a softer, more romantic look, choose pieces in muted colors and lush fabrics. If you want to tap into your darker, more erotic side, seek out a matching set with an open-cup bra and crotchless panty, or a strappy playsuit with brass rings. Whatever you do, take a moment before you present yourself to your lover to dance, prance, or strut, and compliment yourself—in front of the mirror, admiring your physical beauty and sensual boldness. Then, present yourself with confidence!

6. Naughtier Play

Women are becoming increasingly comfortable with exploring Anal Sex (or A-Spot play) as a positive, highly pleasurable element to their sex life. And it makes sense! Your derriere is an erogenous zone, and when approached with open communication (and a lot of lubricant), A-Spot sex can be an exciting and sensual way to play together. Since this kind of stimulation carries a certain element of taboo, it'll make both of you feel a bit wanton and wild, brave, and bold. So if you have a strong sense of intimacy and trust with your partner, go ahead and try it, but together, commit to taking the experience slowly. Ask him to pamper you with an all over sensual massage, caressing and rubbing your cheeks and thighs, making lovely large circles upward, toward your lower back. Allow him to massage your A-Spot externally, with delicate pressure at the opening first. If that feels pleasurable, he could then slide in a finger, and then perhaps a small toy. If your arousal is building and you want to continue, then and only then ask him to insert his shaft—

taking it ever so slowly while continuing to add more lubricant. If you're a beginner, I'd recommend positioning yourself on top first where you'll have the most control over how much you take in. And on that note, if it's your first time, stay on the "shallow side," inserting only the tip of your lover's penis as you begin. Keep breathing and communicating with each other. If at any time you're uncomfortable, just say so! It's your body and your pleasure.

Note: Building up to full A-spot sex is a process, one that can take weeks, months, or years! There is no rush to penetration now, or ever. But there is pleasure to be discovered if you let yourself relax and revel in the sensations of this highly erotic touch.

Remember: Many men enjoy anal stimulation, too! Find out if your man is interested by gently touching his A-spot with the tip of your finger. If he does not discourage you, but instead begins to moan with satisfaction, try inserting a lubricated finger just inside. Again, if he responds positively, continue further until he lets you know when to stop. Take hold of his shaft with your other hand and bring him into your mouth—you are now officially multitasking his manhood!

Want to get even more risqué? You can test your boundaries in other ways by discovering what turns you on beyond your comfort zone. Getting kinky could mean playing with power roles, trading off being dominant and submissive: you could tell him *he's been a very bad boy* and has to pay for it by pleasuring you just the way you like it, or you could surrender to your partner's dominance with handcuffs or silk ties to bind your wrists and ankles to the bedposts. Add in a blind-fold, as removing the sense of sight will heighten all your other senses, making every touch feel *that* much more exciting. Other, bonding-type accessories, like a spanker or a whip made of rubber strands, can stim-ulate the skin too. Whether anal play or light bondage fall into your realm of naughty exploration, be sure to continue communicating all along the way.

7. Take the Orgasm Challenge

When was the time you had two or more orgasms in one Session? (If you answered *yesterday*, consider yourself a unicorn, Mama.) Most women opt for a "one-and-done" approach to orgasms, which is a fine goal, but if one is your *usual,* then going for two (or more!) can be your *something new*. Start by setting an intention that you're going to have an "orgasm marathon" (or at least, two orgasms) because what starts in your mind will take effect in your body. Share this intention with your partner and ready any props or tools you think you'll need—sex toys, lubricant, massage oil, etc. Is there a position that allows you to reach orgasm quickly? If so, do that first. This will give you plenty of time—and stamina—to build up your pleasure once more and reach the sweet abandon of a second, third, even fourth orgasm. Believe that you can do it! Breathe deep and slow into your lower belly to create sensual tension, use your vibrator, squeeze and release your Kegel muscles, and direct your partner in detail on how you'd like to be touched. Notice the differ-ences between your orgasms—was one more powerful than the other? Easier to reach? Did you achieve them through different methods of stimulation? No matter the difference, feel proud and empowered that you pursued more pleasure than usual.

Feeling a Little Timid?

If you're feeling a bit fearful to try out these playful new experiences, that's okay: it just means there is new territory worth exploring! Playing Together shouldn't feel like a scary obligation, so take baby steps and only try things you have an innate curiosity about. This Sexy Session isn't meant to throw you into the deep end, but rather, to get you both to play a little closer toward your edge.

The scenario you choose doesn't *have* to be wild or profound, either. Even a subtle tweak to the routine can be enough to make sex feel a little bit more refreshed. For example, if you usually head to bed naked to initiate sex, trying throwing on a chemise and doing a twenty-second striptease, or maybe you take a little more time for foreplay than usual. Together you'll feel proud to have tried something new and played your way to reigniting your sexual spark. As with all your Sexy Sessions, have a loving chat afterward about your experience, and share the next new scenario you'd like to test out with each other. Make a commitment for more *sexual playtime.*

YOUR SEXY SESSIONS JOURNAL

Now it's time to reflect! Take a moment to recall your playtime session and journal your thoughts; free-form or by answering these questions:

1. How would you describe your Playing Together Session?

2. What new thing did you try? How did you decide on that choice?

_____

_____

_____

_____

_____

_____

3. How did playing a little closer toward your edge feel?

_____

_____

_____

_____

_____

4. What "new thing" would you like to try next?

_____

_____

_____

_____

_____

Make Date Night a Priority

TWO WEEKS AFTER I gave birth to our son, my husband burst through the front door into the living room, proudly holding up two tickets to see the rock band, Muse. "Amazing!" I said. "I love Muse! When's the show?"

"Tonight!" he proclaimed.

"Huh? Wait. What?" I was sure he was going to say it was months away.

Suddenly my engorged breasts began to pulsate as I imagined being away from the baby that night for the first time. I started to stammer, searching for a way out—I mean, we'd only just brought him home! But my resistance was met with an impassioned plea:

"I don't want to become one of those couples who doesn't go out just because we had a baby!" my husband said, as if he were reading my mind.

"I know, I know, I don't want that either! But he's just two weeks old. I'm so, SO tired and my vagina *still hurts!*"

"Please, let's do this! Let's be those parents who stay young and free and fun!" he replied.

He was dead serious, and while I thought he had terrible timing, I appreciated his intention. He didn't want our unique sense of spirited, social fun together to fade away just because we'd become parents.

I understood that, but still, the idea of making any sudden changes to our newfound, nightly baby routine made me panic. I was perfectly satisfied to snuggle up on the couch watching (no, sleeping through) films and eating frozen lasagna brought over by friendly neighbors. Plus, like I said, *my vagina*.

I told him how anxious I was, and so we talked through each concern:

What if the baby needed us?
My mom would stay with the baby and we would keep our phones on.

Where would I pump?
In the car, before and after the show. He'd pack up the cooler.

What if I wanted to leave?
We could leave at any time.

Should I have a beer?
Definitely. My milk supply was high, so I could afford to pump and dump!

With the concert just hours away, I didn't have much time to waffle or debate. So I threw on some lipstick and jumped in the car. I had a beer (the joy!) and I rocked out until I had to sit down and rest my aching ladybits.

Ultimately, was it a little too soon? *Yes.*

Did I limp around like a woman who'd just pushed out a giant baby? *Yes.*

Did we scream at the top of our lungs and make out to our favorite songs? *Yes.*

Did we leave early? *Yes.*

But were we proud that we'd gone on a truly amazing date? *HELL YES!*

We were out of the house and back out in the "real world" together—as lovers! It was as though we made some kind of a symbolic statement to step away from our parenting routine and reinstate our status as a romantic couple.

After my initial resistance, I was so happy I'd said yes to packing up my pump and pads and hitting the show with him. There was a renewed spark between us, reminding us that regular date nights were essential for keeping our relationship alive, youthful, and aroused. That night set the stage for our commitment to keep dating each other, to keep switching up the routine for the sake of romance—despite the demands and duties of parenthood.

When Date Night Dies

As the kids multiply and the exhaustion intensifies and budgets tighten up, date night tends to be the first to fall by the wayside. Here is an all too familiar example from an exasperated husband:

We try to plan a date night all the time, but my traffic-filled commute leaves me feeling completely fatigued by the time I arrive home. When I get there, she's totally frazzled and depleted from the three kids competing for her attention all afternoon: overseeing all their homework, cooking, and cleaning up dinner—and that's all after she's been working herself. So we lose steam and just cancel date night. Weeks have gone by and now months, without a date. We just keep canceling. I say to myself, wait, we used to be the fun couple out of all our friends! But now, we're just so flat. So fatigued. That's just our new routine.

This perfectly exemplifies the problems of the modern couple, making it easier to just say, *Let's just skip date night tonight.*

It's not just exhaustion that causes so many of us to cancel date night, it's a shift in mind-set that goes from *us . . .* to *them.* Think about how life has changed since having kids: Are you constantly planning new and exciting activities for your children and for the family together, but not so much for you and your partner? Therein lies the dilemma.

As parents we fall into a role of *service* to our kids, providing stimulation, steadiness, and security for them. Of course, the children need this! Family life thrives on routine, stability, and safety, but at the same time, we leave the excitement, surprise, and escapism of an active dating life with our partner behind. And that's the juice that keeps you going—it's the gas that fills up your tank as a couple. Prioritizing date nights invites newness, mystery, excitement, and action back into a relationship: all things we need to thrive as a couple with kids.

· · · · · · · · · · · · ·

The true beauty of dating your spouse?
It's just you two, being you two.

· · · · · · · · · · · · ·

If dating is the fuel that reconnects you as a couple to the exciting, refreshing, and interesting, then it's important to go back to playing the dating game. Date night should be used as a tool to experience something wonderful together and learn something new about each other—even if you've been together for many years. It's a tool that enables you to see one another as the sexy, interesting, and independent beings you still are in addition to the amazing parents you've become.

That said, how do you reinstate date night? Here are the five most effective types of dates for breaking up your parental routine and giving your relationship the most bang for your babysitting buck.

1. THE AMAZING DATE

Forget about yet another movie and pizza night at your local go-to spot. The Amazing Date is all about daring yourselves to do something different and adventurous: a wild rock concert, a sexy dance lesson dressed to the nines, or a boozy nighttime river cruise. The whole point is that your shared exploration and discovery can be a huge turn-on. The titillation will begin even before the date gets started! The anticipation alone builds excitement and sparks chemistry, as you ponder the possibilities together while you're getting dressed: *What might happen at this burlesque show? What will we see, smell, feel? Will we be turned on, together . . . in a public space? Will I be pulled up on stage? Will he? What will happen if we cut loose and have two strong cocktails, or even three, at the Silent Disco Party? Will we get sloppy and silly and flirtatious, just like we used to?*

Excitement and uncertainty of what *could* happen are key to rekindling romance and desire. Anticipation is the greatest aphrodisiac of all. Planning an Amazing Date pretty much guarantees that you'll see, feel, and experience something unique, exhilarating, and thought-provoking together, which makes for great conversation about something other than the kids!

> Tip: Conserve energy for your big night out with a midday nap or encourage your partner to take public transportation to avoid feeling drained from sitting in traffic. Think outside the box! Have your sitter come an hour early to cook for the kids and ask her to clean up too. Remember, you want to GO BIG on your Amazing Date, without petering out at ten o'clock!

2. THE STOLEN SUNDAY

Once every six weeks or so, Steal a Sunday: leave the kids in someone else's hands and take the whole day to yourselves as a couple, returning only once the kids are already in bed. (The only challenge is being able to stomach the guilt that will undoubtedly creep up.)

When you take an *entire* Sunday to yourselves, you feel like you've been on vacation. It's *that* rejuvenating. The freedom you'll taste together is staggering, stupendous, and awe-inspiring in comparison to the standard Sunday routine. There's also a hint of rule breaking; of doing something you're not technically supposed to do as parents—and *that* bit of naughtiness can create some serious arousal between you. Because you have the whole day, you can do *so much together:* share a morning workout, have a long brunch, stroll around the shops, visit an art gallery, take a drive, pop into a cooking class, catch a movie, make love in a hotel you rent by the hour. If you're up for it, you could *literally do all of this in one day*, but you can also just do nothing together. You can laze about in the park, with a picnic basket and blanket, listening to music, people-watching, playing card games and napping (yes, napping is totally epic on a date). That's the beauty of a Stolen Sunday without the kids. There's no rushing, no cooking, no carpooling, no kids' birthday parties, no tending to anyone else's needs, no drama while visiting with the grandparents.

It's just you two, being you two.

This is a fantastic break from the familiar. Because family life thrives on stability and routine, each day can start to feel the same, and so your relationship can start to feel the same as well. You know what to expect from each other, from the minute you wake until the moment you go to bed. That kind of monotony can be kind of boring and cause your sex life to turn stale! On the flipside, what fuels an impassioned relationship, year after year, is exactly the opposite: it's mystery, newness, excitement, and unpredictability. A well-curated Stolen Sunday can provide all of that, and more!

No matter how much you value family time on the weekends, or how indulgent this one may feel, I implore you . . . *please, steal a full Sunday every now and again*! Then, bask in the afterglow of the time spent together. If you really can't take the full day, commit to catching at least four hours in morning or afternoon.

3. THAT MORNING MAGIC

If you can't swing childcare for a full Stolen Sunday, or you're often just too depleted in the evenings to motivate for an Amazing Date, then this is the one for you. First, call into work to say you're going to be in two hours late, or if you don't work outside the home, just clear your morning mom agenda. Your partner will do the same. Then, drop the kids off at school or take the baby to the nursery, and then set off together to make a little Morning Magic happen. Do whatever you like: walk to the coffee shop, browse the farmers' market, go back to bed, have a Quickie. Skipping out on work or your usual morning regimen to spend it doing *whatever pleases you both* is just the right amount of rebellion to get you both excited. By cultivating a sense of freedom-to-frolic within the highly structured routine of parenthood, you'll connect to the outside world together, which is an extremely stimulating place—just open your eyes! If you don't do any other "dating" within your marriage, be sure to score some Morning Magic every week. Getting out of the house together reclaims the world as your oyster, providing opportunities to participate in the world together as an active, alive, and engaged couple—not just as partners-in-parenting inside the confines of your home. It's cheap, and it only takes a few hours.

4. THE GROUP GATHERING

Once a month, invite two, three, or four couples over for a Group Gathering. Make it a potluck where everyone brings a dish, or share a list of ingredients for each to bring and you can cook communally while making cocktails and sharing stories and laughter. Turn on music and kick off a dance party, play a provocative card game like Cards Against Humanity or Draw What?!. You're making your own grown-up party, so it's up to you to create the fun! And always be sure to steer the conversation back to adult topics when it ventures into kiddie territory (which, invariably, it always does).

To completely alleviate the financial and logistical stress of everyone finding a babysitter, tell your friends to bring their kids over and that you'll put them in a separate room where they can play, watch a movie, and eat dinner together while the adults socialize. If you want the party to go late, lay out a bunch of sleeping bags and let them fall asleep when they're ready. If the kids are still small and need supervision, hire a junior babysitter (like a teenage neighbor) to keep watch. Everyone can chip in a little cash to contribute to the service!

If you love hosting, claim a Saturday night every month to throw this "parent party" at your place, or suggest a rotating schedule where you alternate houses. If you like theme parties, consider adding one to your Group Gatherings: Fancy Dress, Game Night, Disco Party, etc.

This Group Gathering is a low-cost alternative to a big night on the town, and it effectively says, *we can even have grown-up fun INSIDE the house*, which for parents, many of whom are severely stuck in a domestic routine at home, will feel like a revelation. Plus, it fosters a sense of community within your tribe to get together and cut loose on a consistent basis. As a bonus, you will find yourself more likely to have a romantic rendezvous with your spouse after the party, since you'll be only steps away from the bedroom.

5. THE SEX DATE

Two to three times a year, my husband and I sneak off to a hotel together for a night away from the kids. We call it what it is: a Sex Date. Why? Because *not* having sex at a hotel while you're away from the kids is borderline criminal. There is nothing quite like the fresh, cool, expensive sheets of a beautiful hotel bed, or a sexy soundtrack playing on the sound system. An indulgent dip into the minibar; a long, luxurious bubble bath, and then, an awesome Sexy Session, of course! Most importantly, there's an absence of your usual stress triggers, like a messy house, a pile of bills, a menu to plan, etc. Immersing yourselves in a new environment helps you tune out anxiety and relax. Remember Mama, when you're more relaxed, it's far easier to embrace your sensuality and increase your arousal.

Note: While Sex Dates can be a smashing success, sometimes they carry high expectations to have *the best sex ever.* Instead of feeling any pressure, I encourage you both to keep a sense of humor and allow yourselves to be flexible when things don't go according to plan. For example, I once got pink eye during a Sex Date at a glamorous hotel in Chicago. *Gross.* But we made the best of a bad situation: I wore a satin blindfold and we conjured up some some spicy roleplay!

So, while a Sex Date might not always turn out perfectly, try to relish in the delicious sense of *getting away* together. Luxuriate in a space you don't have to clean yourself, give yourselves permission to sleep in late and be sensually stimulated by your surroundings. If you don't have the budget to get away, stage a Sex Date at home. Send the kids away to their cousin's house for the night, light some candles, and make the most of your kid-free space.

YOUR MISSION: CREATE NEW KINDS OF DATE EXPERIENCES

Are you up for the challenge? Good! Together with your partner, sit down with your calendar and plan out the next few months of dates, scheduling one of each of the date night ideas listed above. That means five dates in three months, which is ambitious but achievable. If you are able to add a few more than that, then please do so!

Have a local cultural guide nearby to thumb through, or surf the internet for listings, concerts, and special events. Talk about your childcare budget and how you can generate more dating dollars. Discuss whether you're

comfortable starting a "kid care collective" with trusted friends, where
you take turns watching each other's kids so that every couple can have
an opportunity to go out on a date. You'll save a fortune on babysitters! If
budget, time, or other unforeseen circumstances prevent you from regularly going on one of these dates, try a Mini Date instead! Ask a neighbor
to watch the kids while you two take a quick walk around the block at
sunrise or a post-dinner bike ride. Stealing even a few date-like moments
together will still give you the grown-up connection time you crave.

Consider these questions in your planning conversation:

What are our dream Amazing Dates?

List the amazing events, places, and activities you'd like to try that would
excite and amaze you.

_____

_____

_____

_____

_____

When can we swing a Stolen Sunday?

Are there any objections that surface for either of you, an inner voice
telling you that you don't deserve the time away from the kids or the
time together?

_____

_____

_____

_____

_____

How often can we make some Morning Magic happen?

Once a month, or maybe even once a week? Discuss how you'll address being late with your respective bosses, or how you'll shift your schedule if you're your own boss.

Where can we go for a seductive Sex Date?

Discuss your budget for a hotel, who can care for the kids, whether you'd prefer room service or if you might want to try a hot new restaurant nearby.

Which friends shall we invite to our Group Gathering?

Brainstorm a theme or menu ideas, and give your friends a heads-up on a date for the first party.

Be sure to plan each date night and lock in childcare well in advance. Let the excitement and anticipation of the soulful and stimulating experience you'll have together start to build. Revel in the anticipation of each upcoming date, each break in routine. Then, stay on top of it! Stage a new planning session every few months so that your dating calendar is always full.

Infuse Every Day with Sexy Stimulation

I **HAVE A HABIT OF** *fondling the carrots at the grocery store.*

Allow me to clarify. Whenever I grocery shop I tend to linger in the produce department, staring at the spectacularly phallic, well-endowed vegetables: the zucchinis, cucumbers, even the eggplants. It's not that I plan on using them as an all-organic sex toy, it's just that they're so . . . fresh, firm, glistening, and healthy. *I can't help but fantasize about passionate sex with a fresh, firm, glistening, healthy hunk of a man.* The produce simply invokes sensual imagery in my mind and arouses my Mojo.

I savor my grocery store fantasies. These risqué reveries give me a tingle down below, awakening both a mental and physical awareness of my sexuality during these otherwise mundane moments of motherhood. My experience in the produce aisle gives me fodder for my fantasies—*cute stock boy takes grocery-shopping mom in Aisle 5, perhaps?*—and renewed inspiration for some Fantasy Fun in the bedroom with my husband. Plus, I always find a cheeky smile creeping across my face later on as I'm peeling carrots for the kids. They don't know why mommy's grinning, *but I do*. What I know for certain is that having a frisky fantasy while picking out vegetables or waiting on line is a whole lot more fun than just running errands on autopilot.

This ultra-simple act of seeking out sensual stimulation in my daily life (and letting my imagination run wild!) has the power to tune me into my Mojo, stimulate my senses, snap me out of the Mom Zone, and remind me that I'm a hot, vital woman—even when I'm standing in the grocery store in my sweatpants.

Get Sex Back on the Brain

Most moms spend our long, busy days thinking about everything *but* sex. *What errand is next?? What the hell am I going to cook for dinner? Why are my thighs rubbing together?* It's no wonder that so many moms have little-to-no sex drive, no desire to seduce or be seduced. It's because sex and sexiness are so *not* a part of your daily thought process! You know it as well as I do: in order to have great sex with the same person, year after year, decade after decade, you've got to nurture your sexual imagination—you've got to get sex back on your brain—every single day.

Prioritizing your sensual imagination is one of the most important shifts you can make to upgrade your sex drive, improve your relationship, and make your entire experience of motherhood a whole lot sexier. And you can start *today*. No props or planning needed!

The secret? Giving yourself permission to notice the sexy inspiration that already exists in your everyday routine—from household chores to running errands, to dropping off the kids at school, taking the train to work, doing laundry, and cooking dinner. The more you bring sexy back to your brain, the more desire you'll naturally begin to feel in your body. In situations where you were previously bored or irritated, you'll soon find yourself fantasizing and privately turned on. The best part? This practice of *noticing* will carry over into *noticing* the sexiness that still exists within the deep familiarity and routine of your relationship, too.

. . . .

Feed your mind daily with fantasy and you'll nourish yourself and your libido.
Seek out sexy stimulation in your everyday life!

. . . .

Here are a few foolproof ways you can light up your mind (and your Mojo!) with sensual stimulation:

1. FIND THE EXTRAORDINARY IN THE ORDINARY

Start noticing the seductive elements you encounter within your daily routine, and allow your mind to wander into a sensual fantasy. Jot down these sexy cues and remember: there is no shame to this game, no thought too dirty *or* tame. Maybe you get turned on by an orchid blooming, as you imagine your own flower blossoming at the touch of a lover. Or, you spot a gorgeous, velvety couch and imagine how the fabric would feel against your naked skin. You might even linger in the scent of rain as it sparks a memory of when you made love outdoors as the heavens poured down. You might walk down the street where an ex-lover lives and let the memories of the eager, ecstatic sex you had with him flood your brain and ignite your body.

A turned-on, sensual mama nurtures her sensuality each and every day. But it takes effort and practice! The best part is there's no limit to what turns you on when you let go and let your imagination run wild.

Here are a couple examples from moms who put this tool into action:

> *"I pass a riding stable on my way to the gym and it got me thinking . . . that men used to get from place to place on horseback. I surprised myself with my next thought, which was 'Gosh, they must've had really strong inner thighs.' Then, my fantasy was off and running! I thought about some half-naked, rustic cowboy type, in worn leather pants and a hat, with thick, strong thighs. Then, I imagined how he would feel on top of me. It seems so silly, but this fantasy was instantly effective in lighting me up, igniting a sense of aliveness, and getting me to think about sex during an otherwise boring drive. It's just a more sensual, playful way of thinking for me . . . and I like it."*—Jessica, mom of 1

> *"Every Friday, the women in my mommy-and-me group meet at the outdoor shopping promenade. We lay out blankets on the grass and let the little ones run around as we talk about mommy stuff, like preschool admissions, sleep schedules, and so on. Today, I found myself distracted by the 'dancing fountain,' something I'd never really noticed before. As the fountain jets erupted in sprays of water, I found myself thinking about orgasms. Fantasizing about the rising tide of pleasure in a body, and about my own body erupting in an orgasm. At first, it felt bizarre and somewhat inappropriate to be having such a sensual thought on such a regular outing with the kids, but it was exciting, and the excitement of that experience lasted the whole day long."*—Libby, mom of 3

2. HIT THE VIRTUAL EYE CANDY SHOP

What's Eye Candy, you might ask? Why, it's those sweet, cheeky images that give us a little tingle inside, a flash of healthy horniness down below. A momentary escape from reality. Eye Candy is a visual cue that turns you on instantly, an image that whispers, *Psst! Yes, you're a mother. Yes, you're a wife. But don't forget you're also a woman with desires!*

You can also practice seeking out sensual stimulation in the privacy of your own home. Got five minutes to spare before you pick up the kids? Stop what you're doing and search the web for some Eye Candy.

Maybe you've got a thing for hot Hollywood-type hunks, so why not search for a few shirtless pictures of them. Or do firemen turn you on? There's *loads* of deliciously cheesy calendars featuring half-naked heroes with their rippling muscles aglow. But don't limit yourself to sexy dudes. A friend sent me the sexiest music video featuring a couple making out, madly. Their palpable passion for one another inspired an epic make-out session with my own husband later that night. I've seen French lingerie commercials that warmed me from the inside out, with not a single male body in sight. Eye Candy comes in all shapes, colors, and sizes. All you have to do is discover what catches your attention and stokes the flame of your desire.

Catching a glimpse of Eye Candy can be the express track to whetting your sexual appetite. It's squeezing in a quick sexual fantasy before the kids wake up from their nap, making your afternoon much more enjoyable. A small dose just might be your saving grace after your favorite shirt gets blasted by a poop explosion. It could even be the spark that ignites you to want to have sex with your spouse that same night!

A virtual Eye Candy moment has the power to *instantly* stimulate your senses and remind you of your sensual vitality as a woman. So instead of getting caught up in negativity on Facebook, or spiraling into competition mode with "fit moms" on Instagram, check out some Eye Candy instead!

YOUR MISSION: PAY ATTENTION TO YOUR TURN-ONS!

Your mission is simple: open your eyes to the turn-ons that surround you in your daily life. They are *everywhere:* the buzzing sounds of the city might remind you of the buzz of your favorite vibrator; the barista who makes your coffee might call to mind the lover who helped you discover your best orgasm. Your sensuality is right there, all around you, begging you to pay attention to it. All you have to do is just open your eyes, and allow yourself to get excited and aroused by letting yourself fantasize. Remember: be silly, have fun with it—and don't censor your thoughts!

Start a list on a notes app on your phone, carry around a small notebook, or use whatever works for you as long as it's accessible throughout the day. Jot down the things you see, hear, smell, and feel that please you and make you feel a little lusty. A turn-on could be anything from an advertisement to a piece of graffiti. It could be the taste of strawberries on your tongue or a margarita rimmed with salt. It could be a hot stranger wiping sweat from his forehead. It could be your delivery guy, or your kid's hot, twenty-something track coach. There are no wrong scenarios here—it's YOUR reverie! If it lights you up, write it down—even if it's not something you think "should" turn you on.

Take your mission a step further and *act on those frisky feelings.* Conjure the fantasy later in the day and initiate a Solo Session, a Quickie, or even a Long Love Session. Your fantasy, your choice!

Getting sex back on your brain is one of the most important shifts you can make to get—and keep—your sensuality burning bright. Noticing—and delighting in—the sensual cues you experience in your ordinary routine can leave you feeling feminine, sparkling, and infused with palpable, turned-on energy, *all day long*. It's a subtle shift you can set into motion that'll create a noticeable difference in how you feel in each and every moment.

So . . . What Turned You On?

As you start seeing your routine world in a sexier way, jot down your thoughts here as a way to validate your experience. As always, you might just surprise yourself with what you've learned!

What did you see that turned you on?

_____

_____

_____

_____

What turn-on(s) surprised you?

_____

_____

_____

_____

Have you noticed any changes in your libido or lustiness?

_____

_____

_____

_____

Do What You Desire

MAMA, YOU'RE SO close to the finish line! You've committed to nurturing the sexy woman that you are, and you've made the practices of self-care and self-pleasure top priorities. So now that you're a pro at honing your sensual desires, it's time to (re)discover what makes you really tick by identifying your passions outside of the boudoir—and then pursuing them. Mastering the art of "doing you" and exploring your personal and/or professional desires are as fundamental to awakening your Mojo as whetting your sexual appetite.

My career as an entrepreneur has always been my passion: a source of excitement, accomplishment, and confidence. Having my own business is an exercise in doing what I desire. In turn, this commitment to doing what I really want to do inspires my sexual desire; by truly owning what I want—be it professional, personal, or otherwise—I feel sexy, alive, and liberated. Having my own ambitions ignites my sense of personal power, keeping my libido lit and inner fire burning bright.

Since having babies, I'll admit that the lines between career and motherhood have often blurred to the point of confusion. While I have the luxury of controlling my own hours, workload, and the amount of time I spend with my family, I still find it difficult to strike a balance. Whenever I give my all to my work, I feel guilty for not giving enough of my time and energy to my family and household responsibilities. On the flip side, whenever I dive into full-on mommy-mode, I judge myself for not "doing what it takes" to further advance my own business. So there they are: my two deepest desires, seemingly at odds with each other forever . . . or so I thought.

My perspective had a major shift when I allowed myself to admit that I am a better mother when I pursue my passions. For many years, an inner voice was nudging me to write this book and share my truth about my personal experience of motherhood, Mojo, and marriage. Yet, I was already feeling pulled apart by horses trying to juggle parenthood with running Booty Parlor. I was already overcommitted and overstretched—how was I going to write a book on top of everything else? But there was no denying my inner voice; that burning desire to write about and share my experiences with other mothers only grew as time went on. I knew I wasn't alone in this struggle; I felt that this book was my highest calling.

I just wasn't sure how I would ever find the time, focus, and discipline to add in yet another big project, to do this thing that I so deeply desired. After starting and stopping the book countless times, I experienced an aha moment: if I wanted to not only dive into this desire but also bring it to fruition, I would have to create the extra time to work on it. That meant I'd have to get up even earlier in the wee hours of the morning. I would also need to discipline myself to go to bed earlier because I knew that come morning the temptation to hit the snooze button would be hard to resist. I would need to channel the fire and passion of that inner voice—the one who was so insistent that I do what I desire—into a consistent rise-and-shine regimen that put me at my desk a full hour before everyone else woke up.

To ensure I maximized that hour and made the most out of the extra time, I set the coffeepot to a timer so that a freshly brewed cup of joe awaited me when I dragged myself out of bed. And there it was: one full hour. Peace and quiet. No distractions. I could stay focused and present, developing my desire and expressing that voice that yearned to be heard. At last, progress! I'll admit that while it wasn't easy to sacrifice an hour of precious sleep, the firm decision to finally start and finish this thing was all I needed to keep me going. Setting this powerful intention for myself to do what I desired was what helped me get the job done. With these newfound five hours a week, the balancing act of mother-hood and my desire no longer felt like a constant battle of competing commitments. Waking up early didn't deplete me, as I worried it might. In fact, quite the opposite happened: pursuing my heart's desire—and actually making real progress on it—turned me on, gave me energy, and freed me from the "I don't have enough time/bandwidth/energy" mind-set that really only drained me before I'd even given it a shot.

The Art of Doing YOU

As mothers, we must give ourselves permission to pursue our passions. As women, we deserve to honor our individuality and creativity, giving our pursuits the time and energy they deserve. Because when we do, we are happier—more satisfied and turned-on—and ultimately, more present, patient, and engaged as mothers. We've stated this before, but let's say it again: What's good for mama is good for the family!

They say that when a child is born, a mother is born. But, sometimes, when a child is born, a hard-earned career gets derailed, an education is halted, projects and passions and hobbies are put on hold, indefinitely. Sometimes, when a child is born, a woman's desires become thrown into confusion—taking a back seat to everyone else's needs but her own.

But Mama, your dreams are not disposable. They are key to your aliveness, and to the return of your Mojo. By taking the time to pursue your passions—*to do what you desire*—you're making a powerful statement that *you* matter. That your desires matter. That you are a mother who adores her children, but knows her own happiness is what's important at the end of the day. Because a happy mama, who is excited about her own life and her own desires, is a mama who can give herself generously and abundantly to the family that she loves.

· · · · · · · · · · · ·

YOUR WANTS, DESIRES, AND GOALS ARE WORTHY.
So . . . *DO WHAT YOU WANNA DO!*

· · · · · · · · · · · ·

Whether you work full-time or part-time, took an extended break from your career when you became a mother, or fulfilled your lifelong ambition by becoming one, we've all taken mothering so seriously at some point that we forgot to tend to our own personal passions, interests, and desires. We convinced ourselves that we didn't have the time for them, or told ourselves we'll make time for them once the kids are older. Why do we do this to ourselves? How can we be expected to nurture our children and families without resentment if we don't take care of our own needs, too?

What if I told you that individuality, self-fulfillment, accomplishment, *and* pleasure are all available to you throughout motherhood? Here are a few simple tips for diving into your desires and getting back to doing YOU:

1. Dive into Discovery

As an empowered mama, you can have, do, and be anything you want. However, you first need to identify what your desires really are. Let's face it: you may not have spent the greatest amount of time and attention on your own personal dreams and wishes since you became a mother. Or maybe you have, but often feel guilty about precious time spent away from your child. Or maybe your truest ambition was to become a mother, but now that the kids are heading into school full time, you're longing to immerse yourself in something new that gives you a sense of purpose. No matter what your unique circumstances are, it's time to dive into discovery and unearth the ambitions, cravings, and passions you most want to explore. Clarifying what you desire is the most important gift you can give yourself! Whether your dreams revolve around a career, creative pursuits, service and charity, hobbies, self-care, travel, fitness, or education, brainstorming and writing them down is the first step toward bringing them to fruition. Dream big and dare to ask yourself . . . *What's possible for ME as a woman?*

Allow your desires to take the wheel as part of your journey to awakening your Mojo. Today is about asking, *What do I want?* instead of, *What should I do next that ensures everyone else's needs are met but my own?*

Read and answer the following questions:

What do you desire to do outside of motherhood?

What's burning in your heart? What idea is circling in your brain, turning you on, absolutely refusing to leave you alone? If you're a working mom, what do you dream of doing outside of work?

Sit for a moment in quiet contemplation and listen to what your intuition is telling you. What does that whisper (or shout) say? Pay attention to sensations that percolate in your body when you consider the possibility of realizing the desires that arise in your mind's eye. Then, make a list of the desires you'd like to pursue that would feed your soul as a woman, inspire a sense of feminine independence, fuel your creativity or professional dreams, and ultimately, reignite your Mojo.

Your list might include anything from *finish my master's degree* to *pick up ballet practice again, launch my own mommy blog, sell my homegrown vegetables at the farmers' market, work as a makeup artist, volunteer at the hospital, learn how to arrange flowers,* or *practice weight lifting three times a week.* Whatever *it* is, it's yours to dive into and discover.

_____

_____

_____

_____

_____

_____

_____

_____

♥ **How do you want to feel about yourself once you're engaged in this new undertaking?**

How do you want to feel as a woman? As a mother? As a partner? For example, you might say, *When I'm playing music again, I will feel like a more expressive, passionate woman—in tune with the raw creativity I know exists within me.* Or, *When I'm hosting jewelry parties, I'll feel like a more confident and equal partner, more self-reliant and independent—earning money and being more social, too.* Or, *When I'm tending to my garden, I'll feel connected to nature, quietude, and beauty. This is the dose of mental calm and clarity I need to feel like a more patient mother.* Or you might just use a handful of words like: *I'll feel sexy. Youthful. Free. Happy. In the flow.*

Write down several statements of how you would like to feel below:

I want to feel . . .

_____

_____

_____

_____

_____

_____

♥ **Are there financial goals or costs attached to your desire?**

If so, what are they? To earn enough to pay for your child's karate lessons? Enough so you can quit your full-time job? Or do you want to build a financial empire that allows you to retire at fifty?

My financial thoughts are:

_____

_____

_____

_____

_____

_____

Note: Try not to put too much financial pressure on yourself during this exercise. Exploring business models, costs, and projections will come later, otherwise, you might wind up discouraging yourself. The point of this initial discovery phase is to focus on which of your desires could generate the most wholeness and happiness, more than say, getting rich. My goal for you is to stake your claim to your personal freedom by pursuing what you are passionate about—and that alone is a true measure of your success.

♥ **What are some first steps you could take to start pursuing this desire?**

For example, if you desire to have a career again, you might connect with another mama who's mastered the juggling act of family and pursuing her professional passions. Ask if she'll be an active mentor to you. Or, if harnessing creativity is your M.O., take a live workshop or online class to deepen your knowledge or skill set of your favorite hobby.

Maybe you're determined to get in the best shape of your life: tour your local gyms looking for a group fitness challenge you could immerse yourself in. If you want to become a marvelous chef, enroll in a digital cooking course and rearrange your kitchen to create a proper workspace. If you used to play the guitar, take it out and dust it off!

Know that right now, you don't need a master plan—just a starting point to taste your desire once again. Beginning to learn or do anything new can be as simple as searching Google or watching instructional videos on YouTube, whatever gets you to actually start your pursuit.

My first steps are:

_____

_____

_____

_____

_____

_____

Note: If your list of desires turns out to be a mile long, take a moment to prioritize which one is calling your name the loudest. Or, if you're coming up blank on your list of desires, don't panic! Give yourself some time to figure out what you really wanna do. Since becoming a mother, your interests may have changed and it may take weeks or months of brainstorming to figure out what it is you want to pursue. That's okay, Mama. Please, give yourself the time and space to do just that.

2. Seek Out Support

Now that you have a vision for what you want to do, proclaim it out loud and share with your nearest and dearest. Tell your girlfriends. Your spouse. Your kids. Make a choice in how you will speak about this new "thing" that you want to make a reality. Speaking about it in a positive, passionate, and confident way will help strengthen your belief that it's possible; that you deserve to do this thing you so desire. And, yes, you might be afraid to speak out in this way and feel totally vulnerable. You may have forgotten just how capable you are of trying something new— of stepping outside your comfort zone, of working toward a personal goal. But guess what, Mama, you can do it! And speaking about it with intention is going to help you get there. The great Sufi poet Hafiz wrote, "What you speak becomes the house you live in." So if you've been saying *I'm lost*, try turning that around and saying *I'm finding myself.* If you've been saying *I can't,* now try saying *I can do anything.* Instead of saying *I'm bored*, say *I'm excited to try something new*!

As you begin voicing your most heartfelt desires, consider who's available to support, inspire, and hold you accountable. Mentors, colleagues, your family and friends, maybe even that entrepreneurial mom whom you've always admired. Who's been through what you're going through, who's achieved what you want to achieve? Who can help cover the kids for a couple hours while you do *you*? Enlist them in your personal support group and invite them to have your back. Remember: Those who love and respect you will *want* to help you so don't be shy about asking.

Most importantly, share your excitement with your spouse and call upon him for support. Your partner *wants to* see you feeling turned on, alive, and excited about your own life! Communicate that you need to have some time and space to be free and to be *yourself*. Let him know that you'll need his help with kid duty or with helping you find alternative childcare if he's not available. If he feels threatened or hesitant about you exploring your passion, assure him that you're not abandoning him—and that your desire to do something else doesn't diminish your desire to be with him. All you're asking for is his help so that you can create the time to do whatever you choose to do in order to be the person you've always wanted to be. Then, ask him how you can support him in doing the same. This is an opportunity for each of you to honor your independence, recognizing that you both deserve the freedom to be your own self. This healthy acknowledgment of your individuality is separate from your role as mother and his as father—and can be a big turn-on in the bedroom. Breaking out of the codependent zone will give both your libidos a boost because you're celebrating the unique qualities about the other person that drew you together in the first place.

3. Take the Time

Who among us doesn't feel like we're short on time and behind on our endless to-do lists, yes? And yet, we all have the power to shift our perspectives from *I have no time* to *I will make the time*. Whatever this thing is that you wanna do is going to rejuvenate your soul, give you a jolt of inspiration, and raise up your libido, reminding you that you are more than just a mother. Whether you're starting a blog, becoming a yoga instructor, taking a night class, or launching a new business idea, you'll probably need anywhere from two to four hours a week just to get the ball rolling. Yes, you're going to have to discipline yourself to stay on track, devoting your time and energy to stay on schedule with no excuses. Determination and work ethic are nonnegotiable in the quest to doing what you wanna do. But once you start doing it, I promise you'll not only have more energy to keep going, but you'll also commit to taking the time to do it, no matter how busy you are.

Here are a few ways to carve out those two to four hours per week for yourself:

Turn Wasted Time Around Spend a few days tracking your time to see clearly where your time is being spent, and where it's being wasted. Write down everything you're doing and how long each activity takes you. Then, look for obvious windows where you're wasting time. Do you spend half the baby's naptime scrolling through social media? Or, do you become a complete couch potato once the kids are in bed, and realize that you're spending about three hours in doing so? Notice if you're doing a little bit of laundry every day, and ask yourself if you could consolidate that task to two days a week instead. Once you've logged a few typical days on paper, add up all that "wasted" time. There's a good chance you just might surprise yourself and discover at least a few hours that could be better spent in pursuit of your desires.

Wake Up Early For sleep-deprived mamas, suggesting an *earlier* wake-up call could feel like a slap in the face. But the wee hours of the morning when everyone else is still sleeping is the ideal time to do whatever it is you wanna do. Just think about it: if you woke up at five a.m. instead of your usual six a.m., you could score five whole hours per week to pursue your passions. I recommend easing your way into an earlier wake-up call, setting back your alarm a little bit each week, slowly increasing your me-time. If you can't bear the thought of waking up earlier every single day, try committing to it just two to three days per week. The beauty of the early bird approach is that not only does it give you uninterrupted time to work on whatever pleases you, but you're also making yourself your first priority of the day. Putting yourself first will help you to continue meeting everyone else's needs throughout the day without feeling deprived or resentful.

Say No to More Consider what you can start saying *No* to in order to clear your schedule and create more time to pursue your passions. Are you overcommitted to too many engagements at your kids' school? Are you running too many errands for your sister-in-law? Have you taken on an unnecessary extra project at work that's keeping you late at the office too often? And, counterintuitive as it may seem, are you working out so much that you don't have enough time to fulfill this new desire? Trying to squeeze in your fitness routine, domestic duties, *and* your passions all in one day might be too much and quickly lead to burnout. You may need to scratch one or two extraneous engagements from your week in order to make time to pursue the other things that will actually feed your soul.

Note: If you're a mom who works a full-time job, finding the time *and* energy outside of work hours and family time might seem impossible. But I assure you, it's not! Consider how you might *do what you wanna do* on your lunch hour, or how you might be able to carve out vacation time for a solo trip to catch your favorite motivational speaker, or spend time in a cabin somewhere off the grid working on your art.

4. Embrace Your Ego

The ego typically gets a bad rap, but sometimes it's there to teach us something. During the course of writing this book, I often woke up in a cold sweat, terrified, horrified, and paralyzed with fear. *Who was I to write this book? Who wants to read advice from me? Can I publish this if my sex life is a work-in-progress myself? Is my post-baby brain sharp enough to even get this done?* Ah, there she was again: my inner critic. For as long as I can remember, this critic (who I often call my evil twin) has chased after me, shouting at me to work harder, do better, and achieve more. She has effectively motivated me to move toward my goals and desires, but at the same time, delivers a particularly heavy-handed dose of fear and crippling self-doubt. She wields a double-edged sword, that one.

No one said that following your dreams during motherhood was going to be easy or that the transition of stepping into your truth would be a smooth one. When we have the courage to follow our desires, it's as though we automatically open the door for self-doubt, guilt, and self-sabotage to come marching through.

What you need to do, Mama, is: Shut. That. Door. To pursue your desires, you must absolve yourself of fear, or at least learn how to tolerate it when it creeps up. Remember, what doesn't kill you makes you stronger. You must face your ego head-on from more of a detached place, squandering negativity and anxieties with positive affirmations. Something like, *Mama, you got this. Woman, you were born to do this! Babe, just try it and see what happens!* Forget about what your own evil twin thinks, and just keep showing yourself that you are capable by continuing to put one foot in front of the other.

Tip: Confront your internal naysayer with positive reminders of how smart, capable, and powerful you truly are. Remember, your interests, passions, and needs outside of motherhood are just as important as everyone else in your household. Guilt will challenge that; it will tell you that you're not doing enough, that the time you take for your own desires is time you should be dedicating to your family, your responsibilities, your to-do list. Don't listen to that voice! Acknowledge it, and then tell it to kindly f*ck off. Adopt this mantra: *Guilt is a wasted emotion*—and put that on repeat!

5. Turn Desire into Drive

You've lined up your support network. You've shushed your inner critic and abandoned your guilt. Now, it's time to take action!

Commit to taking small, consistent steps toward doing what you wanna do, several times per week. Don't overthink it, just start doing it. That may mean you carve out three, hour-long working sessions per week to write your book, or work on designing the line of purses you've long wanted to produce. Or, you commit to a six-month yoga teacher training program that requires just three hours a week, and you organize childcare in advance for every single session so that you never miss a class.

Then once you've gotten the ball rolling, nurture your passions with consistency. Goals require patience, focus, and persistence, even if that comes in small, one-hour increments. Yes, progress may come slower than you'd like at this rate, but it's these little doses that will add up over time to become the blossoming change you desire. Make the most of the time you've set aside by ridding yourself of distractions: turn off your phone, log out of social media, lock the door if you need to, and be sure the sitter knows to keep the kids away from you for the duration.

All I ask of you, Mama, is that you try to enjoy doing what you've chosen to do. Even if it's hard! Even when the guilt creeps in. Even if you'd rather be napping. Even if it challenges parts of your brain or body that haven't been used in years . . . just don't complain about it. Savor every moment instead. Squeeze out every last drop of enjoyment, pleasure, and power from the fact that you are *doing what you desire*. Release yourself from any worries or fears surrounding expectations about *the results*. If you allow frustration and fear to seep into the experience, you might ultimately give up. At the same time, know that you'll stop and start, and that there might be plenty of confusion, anxiety, and frustration. Just trust in yourself and your desires and KEEP DOING IT ANYWAY. The only way to build confidence is to do the thing that you're most afraid of doing.

Once you've done that *thing you wanna do,* celebrate your wins, however big or small. Did you whip out two whole blog posts in just under an hour? Hooray! Or maybe just two whole sentences? Hooray, *still*! The goal in practicing your desires is the sheer joy it brings you, not in achieving perfection. The more you lift yourself up with positive reinforcement and pat yourself on the back for even the most insignificant of wins, the more you'll be inspired and motivated to keep it up.

YOUR MISSION:

Mama, your mission is simple: JUST DO WHAT YOU WANNA DO. Take the leap and unapologetically express the authentic aspects of yourself: your talents, passions, interests, and desires. No longer will you ignore or overlook this desire to do *you*, so that you can do *more for your family*. No longer will you let self-doubt or mommy guilt keep you from filling your cup. As a sexy, self-confident mama whose Mojo is now fired up and flowing, there's no more hiding who you are or what your heart desires. This is how you honor yourself as a woman and how you'll continue to stoke the flames of your awakened sensuality. Start doing the things YOU love to do and watch as you become the best mama and partner you're capable of being.

Spontaneous Sex
A Sexy Session

YOU'VE REACHED YOUR final Sexy Session! If you've been following them as I've prescribed then I know you've already generated more frequency, variety, and passion within your sex life.

Yet, it's often at this point in the makeover that some moms start thinking, *Oh, crap! What have I done? Now my partner's making passes at me every day.* While taking the initiative to have better sex with more frequency and feeling has worked to reignite the spark between you, it's also possible that it's sent a message that you're up for it more often than you actually are.

As a result, you might fall back into old patterns. You could start rejecting his advances. Pushing him away. Focusing only on the planned and scheduled Sessions, but neglecting to make room for spontaneity within your sex life. But Mama, if this is the case, then you're missing the point! The reason why we practice and enjoy *scheduled* sex is in order to regenerate an authentic desire and willingness to have *spontaneous* sex!

Here's an example: One night, I was relaxing on the couch after dinner as I often do. The kids were finally quiet in their beds, and all I wanted was giant bar of chocolate and my favorite TV show. My husband sat down next to me and started rubbing my feet. Wonderful, yes, but I was suspect. I wasn't even remotely in the mood. Moments later, he started seductively nuzzling my neck. *Ugh. I knew this was coming.* To myself, I thought, *We've already had our "sex for the week"! Two amazing scheduled Sessions! Isn't that enough?*

My inner voice exclaimed *NO!* before I'd even really taken the time to consider his invitation for sex. I let out a big, disapproving sigh at his advances, and so he stood up and promptly left the room.

Oh no. *I'd rejected him.* I dismissed his attempt at spontaneity and connection, and lost an opportunity to emotionally and physically align with my man. In that instant, I realized I needed to practice what I preach and embody the very philosophy I share with so many other mamas. For a moment, I'd forgotten that the purpose of the Sexy Sessions is not only to rebuild intimate sexual connection—but also to recreate a sense of sexual spontaneity instead of scheduled rigidity! It wasn't a matter of just giving it to him because he wanted sex, but more so, I needed to make an effort and meet him halfway so that we wouldn't fall back into old patterns again. So, I asked myself, *Why was my first reaction a big, fat NO? Is this TV show so important that I can't take a break from it for fifteen minutes? Do I feel ill? Am I irritated with him for any legitimate reason?*

I turned inward and saw that my rationale for such an automatic no was this: *laziness.* I could always just record the show, I wasn't sick. I wasn't angry with him. I reminded myself that I enjoy having sex with him—and that an orgasm is *always worth having,* but I was blocking myself.

I saw two choices: I could stay on the couch and tell him I was just too tired that night and offer him a rain check. I knew he would have been fine with that, since he's not one to hold grudges. Or, I could put down the remote, drop my dress, and take a leap into sexual spontaneity and pleasure with the man I love. And so I did. I tossed my dress at him and frolicked naked down the hall into the bedroom. We jumped onto the bed, wrestling and kissing our way into what turned out to be a delightful and satisfying Session of Spontaneous Sex.

I chose spontaneity over routine. I chose rich, hot intimacy over emotional distance. I chose to orgasm instead of numbing out in front of a screen. I fell back into love and lust that night for the millionth time since we met. Because every time I'm willing to *say yes,* I'm always reminded of just how good sex can be—of how healing it can be to leave everything behind and allow yourself to be swept away into seduction. This is the path to a passionate marriage—always coming back to each other, and always committing to reigniting the passion that brought you together in the first place. Plus, the chocolate and TV were *still* waiting for me afterward.

What I know is this: Prioritizing and planning intimacy provides our sex life with consistency and satisfaction. Whenever we encounter a dry spell, I know I can always count on the twice-a-week Sexy Sessions method to help guide us back toward rich sexual fulfillment. But I don't want a sex life that is only penciled into my calendar. I want an intimate connection that has freedom and flow.

Sexy Session #8: Spontaneous Sex
You've planned sex. Had Quickies. Set aside time for Fantasy Encounters and Receiving Pleasure. You've prioritized, planned, and followed-through, just as you promised you would. **You've made sex an *event* in your relationship, and it's lit up your sex life and reawakened your romantic connection**.

But now it's time to experience the unplanned adventure of Sponta-neous Sex. To *just do it*, on a whim, because you love your spouse—and you love that your pussy feels awake and alive again, just like in the early stages of your relationship.

The beauty of this Session is that there are no rules. No instructions to follow, no games to play or sex dice to roll (unless you choose to!). Once you've said *yes* to the invitation, the only goal is to **make love like you mean it.**

Spontaneous sex could be in the early morning before the kids are up, or at midnight when the house is quiet. *Both are awesome.*

A quick romp while dinner is in the oven and they're occupied with their homework. *Thrilling.*

A sweet cuddle in the kitchen that turns into something much more? *Why not!*

Spontaneous Sex has the power to bring back the feel-good memo-ries of how you felt in the early hot-and-heavy stages of your courtship, when you were lit up with lust, and you couldn't keep your hands off each other. Having Spontaneous Sex says, *I choose you, right NOW.* Not, *I feel obligated to have sex with you only on the days we plan for it.*

There is bravery in the willingness to drop what you're doing for the sake of love and pleasure; a sense of wild abandon and youthful freedom that you will both feel in return.

· · · · · · · · · · · · ·

Saying *Yes!* to Spontaneous Sex makes you
an *active, participating player in your sex life.*

· · · · · · · · · · · · ·

YOUR MISSION: SAY *YES* TO SPONTANEOUS SEX

Your mission is simple: say *YES* to Spontaneous Sex and make love like you mean it. Below are a few tips to practice the art of impromptu intimacy.

1. COMMUNICATE TO GET IN SYNC

As with all your Sexy Sessions, you want to set yourselves up for satisfaction by talking about it. Yes, yes, I know—isn't this Session supposed to be completely *spontaneous*? It is! But it's also okay to have a preemptive conversation that lays out when you might be most receptive to saying *YES* to his advances of spontaneous sex, or him to yours. Is it after all the kids' toys have been put away and you've had a chance to shower and shave so that you feel pretty? Or is it on Sunday when the kids are at Grandma's, after you'd had the opportunity to exercise? It's probably not on the night of your favorite TV show, or just when you've started folding the laundry. Give him some clear examples of when it's the right (and the wrong) time to make a move. And ask your partner to do the same for when it's your turn to initiate! Maybe he needs more time than you think to decompress after work. Or he's too grumpy for sex when his team loses the game, or too tired after he's had the kids all afternoon. Remember, Mama, just like you, there are times when your man just isn't in the mood.

2. PREPARE YOURSELF TO SAY YES

While it may sound counterintuitive, preparing your mind, body, and environment for seduction will help you feel ready to go whenever the invitation arises. For example, notice all the sexiness that exists in your daily life and allow yourself to drift into a mini-fantasy. Squeeze in a Sexy Dance Break, and lay your hands on your body as you do hip circles. Sit for ten minutes in a Sensual Daydreaming meditation. Have a quick Solo Session, and believe that your body *wants* to rise to the occasion of a second orgasm on any given day. Clean up the kid clutter in the bedroom, and set flameless candles to a nightly timer so the mood naturally shifts to something more seductive without you having to think about it. Always make sure your vibrators are charged and that there's a fresh bottle of lubricant near your nightstand. Any and all of these efforts will get your sensuality radiating at a higher level, warming your body and ever so subtly inspiring desire and building authentic arousal. When you fill your mind and sensual space with provocative suggestion, it's more likely your libido will begin humming and your willingness to say *Yes* will increase. Obviously, have some kind of birth control method in place so that you don't have to worry about contraception when the opportunity for Spontaneous Sex arises, unless, of course, you want another baby.

3. REQUEST AN INVITATION

This week, request that your partner initiates this Session, and commit to saying *Yes* when he does. Remember, you're not just saying *Yes* to him to meet your sexual quota or fulfill the requirements of this program. *This is not the case.* You're saying YES to YOU. To pleasure. To play. To orgasm. To living your life as a spontaneous, sensual woman. To being an active, alive, participating player in a sex life that has found its flow again—despite the constant challenges and distractions that come with parenting.

Sure, all this "saying yes!" is great in theory, right? But many mamas tell me that they need *much more* from their partner's initiation style to get their Mojo rising. They tell me that having their breasts groped out of the blue isn't enough for them to generate an enthusiastic *Yes*, or that raising his eyebrows and saying "hubba-hubba" doesn't exactly get them racing into the bedroom, tearing their clothes off in a fit of passion. We need more stimulation, and romance, more investment in our arousal. So, ask yourself this: **What kind of initiation would move you to drop what you're doing and get busy in a split second? What would incite your instantaneous attraction to your partner, so much so that you simply couldn't resist the opportunity to make love?**

You have to figure that out and then tell your partner. Maybe you need them to woo you with interest in how your day was, then offer a deep neck massage and pour you a glass of wine before they make a move. Or maybe you need a text in the morning with a description of what he'd like to do to you when he comes home on his lunch break, bringing you flowers upon his arrival. Or maybe you're the kind of mama that needs him to take charge of cleanup after dinner and send you off to relax with some lingering kisses. Your task is to think about what would help drive your *Yes* and then communicate it to your partner. It takes real bravery to speak your truth, but you deserve an initiation that is worthy of dropping what you're doing in the moment and responding with an enthusiastic *Hell Yes!* By the same token, your partner deserves to know what it takes to turn you on to an awesome Session of Spontaneous Sex.

4. . . . OR TAKE THE LEAD!

You may decide you'd like to be the one to commence a Spontaneous Session. You might prefer to be in control and have the ability to fully prepare for your pleasure. Great! Take the lead and initiate a Spontaneous Session with your partner. A note: With all your newfound Mojo, it's no longer adequate to just say, "So, ummm, should we do it?" Instead, grab your partner, plant a deep kiss on him, and say, "I want you. I want to make love. Let's go." If you prefer to be less vocal in your initiation, start touching yourself while you're lying next to each other in bed. Or, try opening your iPad and pressing play on a sexy porn clip. Better yet, slip off your undies in the car on the drive home from a date and place them in his hand. He'll get the message.

If initiating this Session feels a bit too challenging to you, it's okay. Trust yourself—you have all the tools and motivation you need now. But don't wait until you're burning hot with desire to put the moves on him. Call upon your newfound willingness to *pursue* desire, to be curious about waking your body up, and to investigate what might happen.

5. MAKE LOVE LIKE YOU MEAN IT

Now that you've both said *Yes,* surrender your body and mind to the experience by being fully in the moment with your partner. Being sexually present—and vulnerable—together is one of the greatest opportunities to build intimacy and trust in your relationship. When you allow yourself to be in the moment with your lover (letting go of worry, petty grudges, and negative body banter), sex becomes a shared experience of discovery, expression, and play, allowing you to give and receive nonjudgmental love and pleasure. When you allow everything else to fall away and really tune in to the spontaneous experience that is unfolding right in front of you, you're able to see your partner as a primal sexual being—as your *lover,* and as who he truly is underneath it all. He's no longer just your partner-in-parenting, he's your soulmate again—the person you fell madly in love with. Your partner will see *you* in this very same way. A present sexual connection can alleviate the exhaustion of parenting, wash away the resentment, and banish the boredom that's crept into your bedroom. It's the sweetest honey a Sexy Session has to offer!

To make love like you really mean it, trust your instincts. Go slow or make it kinky. Or make it sweetly seductive, heated loving—even *dirty.* Be as present as possible, pausing to connect to your senses and then following the sensations wherever they want to lead you. What are you tasting? Smelling? Seeing? Feeling? Your lover's feather-like touch tracing down your back? His flesh against your hands as you passionately pull him closer to you? *Be there* in each instant; look deeply into each other's eyes. Explore every part of your partner's body, trying out different kinds of stimulation and witnessing his reactions. Throw your head back and inhale more pleasure into your pelvis. Allow yourself to moan and express your bliss. Say *I love you,* and then whisper something raunchy into each other's ears.

With this Session, place your focus on the journey, not the destination. There's no pressure to explore another reverie from the Fantasy Fun list you made, or make love for a full thirty minutes. There's no need to make sexual history with this one, or to outdo all your other experiences! It could mean you have a marathon make-out session, or that you give and receive oral pleasure. Or maybe you just wind up rubbing your bodies together for a few minutes.

The goal of Spontaneous Sex is to embrace the excitement of impulsivity. To *not* fake passion, but to let it authentically rise between you. To shed any remaining self-consciousness you're holding onto about your body, and to just go for it and witness each other in the moment.

BONUS TIP: How to Take a Rain Check

There will always be times when a *Yes* just doesn't work for you—and that's totally fine! The key is to still say *yes,* but to also say you'll take a rain check. You don't want your partner to feel undesired and rejected, which may lead to another dry spell because eventually he'll stop trying. *Let's not go there.* So on the occasions where you can't reach your *Yes,* (i.e., you ate too much, you have a heavy period, you're rushing to meet a deadline for work), you can say something like: *"Babe, I love these kisses, but I need to prepare for my meeting. Will you ask me again tomorrow?"* Or, *"Yes, baby, I'd love to, but maybe not tonight. Ask me again on Thursday when the kids are at rehearsal!"* This "soft rain check" approach works to reduce any feelings of dismissal and will help balance things out when your sex drives aren't always in sync.

O-NOTES: KEEP A SEXY SESSIONS JOURNAL

Once you've welcomed Spontaneous Sex, jot down your thoughts about the experience:

1. What were your examples of "good times to initiate" and how did you communicate them to your partner? How did he respond? Was he surprised?

_____

_____

2. How did you prepare yourself to say *Yes*? Which tools did you try throughout the course of your daily routine that helped you percolate with passion?

_____

_____

3. What was it about your partner's initiation that moved you to *make love like you mean it?*

_____

_____

4. If you chose to initiate, why? How did it feel? Did being in control allow you to enjoy the experience more?

_____

_____

5. What was the highlight of your lovemaking? Describe the energy.

_____

_____

6. What does it feel like to come back together in an unplanned, impromptu way?

_____

_____

7. After putting in all the work you have, has your chemistry begun to feel more natural? More energized? More intuitive?

_____

_____

· · · · · · · · · · · ·

Your Mommy Mojo Makeover is percolating now, bubbling over with arousal and excitement. There's no question about it, Mama, you're lit up from all the hard work you've been doing, glowing from the inside out because of it. You're dripping with sex appeal, feeling more feminine, free, sexy, and alive than maybe you have in a long time. I don't doubt that you're already seeing the results in your sex life and authentic connection to your partner, too. So why stop there! Let's finish this off with some soul-searching and self-congratulations, as well as a maintenance plan to ensure you keep that Mommy Mojo flowing!

· · · · · · · · · · · ·

Mojo
For Life

Journal It Out

Okay, Mama, let's pause for a moment to reflect on how far you've come. This exercise is an easy journaling session, where you'll review and take credit for all of your sexy accomplishments. If you haven't fulfilled certain goals, this activity will help pinpoint the areas that still need a bit of tuning up. From there I'd recommend going back into the tools for review, and retrying the exercises you've yet to master.

Just sit back, grab a glass, light a candle, and find a quiet, kid-free spot to relax while you answer the questions below. Think back on the amazing things you've done that perhaps you never thought you would want to do, *could* do—or even dare to try!

When we take the time to review our hard work and progress toward something we care about deeply—like ourselves and our relationships—it gives us a sense of empowerment and ownership over our lives and how we live them. You've taken full control of your happiness, sensuality, and confidence, and you're inspired to keep your precious love connection with your partner burning bright, despite the challenges that modern life and parenthood present to you both. So go ahead, give yourself some credit for the newfound sensuality and sexy hot swagger that's emerged!

Answer the following questions to see where you stand. Remember, there are no wrong answers!

1. MAKEOVER MUSINGS

What were your favorite moments during the makeover? Why?

_____

_____

_____

_____

What were your least favorite moments, or the most uncomfortable challenges that arose during the process?

_____

_____

_____

_____

_____

Which Mommy Mojo Block resulted in the biggest breakthrough? Where do you still feel stuck?

_____

_____

_____

_____

_____

2. EMBRACING YOUR BODY

Which parts of your body have you become more accepting of? Have you fallen back in love with a certain part of you that changed dramatically after giving birth?

_____

_____

_____

_____

Are there still parts of yourself that you're beating up? Where are you still stuck? What's holding you back from fully embracing them and showering them with sexy self-love?

_____

_____

_____

_____

Which tools will you continue to practice when your inner critic returns with more nasty negative body banter?

_____

_____

_____

_____

3. EMBODYING SENSUALITY

How has the makeover affected your relationship with yourself? Do you feel more confident? More sensual? More empowered to put yourself, your needs and desires out there?

_____

_____

_____

_____

_____

In what ways have you stepped into your sensual power as a mother, woman, and partner?

_____

_____

_____

_____

_____

Are you actively thinking more about sex and sensuality now that the makeover is almost complete? Which exercises or tools really flipped on the switch that made you see and feel the "sexy" in your daily life? Has your daily "mom routine" become more fun and even flirtatious because of it?

_____

_____

_____

_____

_____

Do you feel more sexually confident now that you've embraced your Sexual Superpower?

_____

_____

_____

_____

_____

Have your overall orgasms and sexual satisfaction improved?

_____

_____

_____

_____

4. SEXY SELF-LOVE

What role did self-love play in your life before the Mommy Mojo Make-over? Where did you place yourself on the priority list?

_____

_____

_____

_____

How important is sexy self-love in your life today, now that you've been practicing the tools?

_____

_____

_____

Have you taken ownership in carving out more me-time and self-care? What did you discover was your best trick to secure that time for yourself? What obstacles are still in your way to claiming that as a part of your daily life?

_____

_____

_____

_____

_____

5. CONSCIOUS COMMUNICATION

Describe any changes in the ways you communicate with your partner about sex and your desires.

_____

_____

_____

_____

With your new communication skills, have you been able to get more of what you want—both in and out of the bedroom—by expressing yourself?

_____

_____

_____

_____

Are there any desires you still feel uncomfortable expressing? How could you approach that conversation?

---

6. RELATIONSHIP REFLECTIONS

How has the makeover affected your relationship outside of the bedroom? Is there more flirtation? More openness and vulnerability? More enthusiasm for each other?

Did practicing the W-words (and embracing Daddy Style) help to reduce the resentment you felt toward your spouse? What other practices could you try to release any residual grudges and irritation?

What changes have you made to bring some magic back to your "dating life"? How is the way you communicate different now? Do you appreciate each other more?

_____

_____

_____

_____

_____

7. SEXY SESSION ASSESSMENT

What was your overall experience like with the Sexy Sessions? Which Sexy Sessions were your biggest wins? Your most difficult stumbling blocks?

_____

_____

_____

_____

_____

Did you try each and every Session? Did you find a favorite and repeat it? Did tackling risqué explorations (like fantasies or mutual masturbation) give you a solid sense of rekindling your desire? Why?

_____

_____

_____

_____

_____

What is your biggest takeaway from practicing this kind of "intimate homework" with yourself and your spouse?

_____

_____

_____

_____

_____

If you and your partner were to make a commitment to keep up with this practice moving forward, what would make sense? Two Sessions per week? Two Sessions every ten days?

_____

_____

_____

_____

_____

8. AND FINALLY . . .

What would you tell yourself at the start, if you knew what you know now about this sensual journey?

_____

_____

_____

_____

_____

By now your confidence and sense of accomplishment must be swelling! May these journal entries become a keepsake that you can look back on for inspiration—and a reminder that you can create positive changes in your life and relationship, and amplify your experience of sensual motherhood! You *can* do that hard work (and play!) to overcome the Mojo Blocks and challenges that will undoubtedly arise. The evidence is right here in your answers!

Your Mommy Mojo Maintenance Plan

Congratulations, you've done it! You completed the Mommy Mojo Makeover.

You embarked on a journey into becoming the most fun, sensual, confident, and satisfied version of your hot mama self. You rediscovered a reenergized and sexier emotional and physical connection to your spouse. You made your daily "mom routine" more fun and flirtatious, you scored more me-time, and carved out more space for your desires, dreams, and interests as a woman. You explored and practiced new tools and techniques to propel your sex life beyond the frustration and monotony that creeps into most long-term relationships with children.

I hope you are inspired by your own willingness to grow, and your bravery to communicate your deepest desires within your relationship. This is only the beginning of a domino effect that will inspire your partner to grow and change alongside you.

This process has been about giving yourself permission to develop and express your sensuality as an integrated part of motherhood. This was your odyssey to illuminate how sex and sensuality could play a part in your life as a mom and woman, and contribute greater happiness, satisfaction, and growth in your relationship.

It doesn't stop here, Mama. Your Mojo is your saving grace; an inspiring, creative, nurturing, loving power source to call upon time and time again—no matter how hectic and demanding your life may be. When you feel like the sexiest, most fabulous, and vibrant version of you—confident, dedicated to self-love, and in hot pursuit of sexual satisfaction—it creates a ripple effect on your life. With all this newfound Mojo, you naturally feel less stressed and more energized; you have more personal freedom and feel less burdened by your responsibilities. All around, you've become a happier woman, a more present and patient mother, and, of course, a much more satisfied spouse.

You don't want to wind up back where you started and find yourself once again stuck in the Mom Zone: exhausted, resentful, unfulfilled, and experiencing unsatisfying sex. That's why you're going to need a Mojo Maintenance plan! These suggestions will help keep your Mojo in line:

1. SCHEDULE MOJO MOMENTS INTO YOUR LIFE

For all of us busy mamas, scheduling in Mojo Moments is the only way to ensure we stay on point with our Mojo goals. It's easy to slide into old habits like scrolling through Facebook or picking up toys when we come across even just a brief moment of free time. But those things do nothing for your Mojo! Take a good look at your schedule for any windows of free time and then use your favorite makeover tools and activities to inspire short snippets of Mojo Moments.

If you have five minutes, throw on a pretty bra and lacy panties and connect to yourself in the mirror. Swipe on some lip gloss and allow your mind to drift toward thoughts of your spouse dipping strawberries in chocolate and feeding you. Imagine how the warm chocolate will taste, and even lick your lips as you imagine it. Grab your favorite vibe and indulge in a quick Solo Session.

If you have ten minutes, squeeze in a mini Mommy Pop-Out. A walk around the block *by yourself* can still be the break you need to snap you out of the Mom Zone and help you reenergize for a Quickie once the kids are asleep.

If you have one hour, seize it! Write that blog post you've been talking about for months, or race outside to train for the 5K race you and your bestie had promised to do. Or, have a Solo Session and take a nap!

In addition to creating these mini Mojo Moments, keep up with planning Date Nights, Moms' Nights Out, and Pop-Outs. Book your childcare well in advance. Make your Mojo plans and stick to them!

2. LOVE AND CARE FOR YOURSELF

By now, you should be tuned in to your negative body banter habits. And since you're now more aware of them, you can catch them as they're happening and turn them around with ease. Don't spiral backward into beating up your thighs, bust or belly! Lay on the positive, sexy self-love affirmations real thick.

Set up affirmation reminders or alarms on your phone, perhaps to some inspiring music. Seeing a loving message to yourself on your phone like, "Hey, Sexy Mama!" or, "Your ass looks amazing today, Mama!" will bring a smile to your face and reinforce what you already know about yourself—that you're one hot mom. Yes, it's a little silly, but who cares if it gets the job done? The same goes for your self-care rituals. Check in with your Self-Care strategy list that you made. Are you giving yourself what you promised you would? Eating right? Sleeping enough? Saying no? Practicing yoga? Make a concentrated effort to weave in self-care each and every day—no excuses. If you see your fellow mamas beating up their bodies or not getting enough me-time, share the tools you've learned with them as your own.

3. PRIORITIZE YOUR SEXY SESSIONS

For the last four weeks, you've found a steady groove with two Sexy Sessions a week. You've explored variety, daring play, and creative, communicative pathways to experience more pleasure with yourself and your spouse. So . . . where do you go from here? It's up to you and your partner to work together as a team and decide how to keep the Sexy Sessions running like a well-oiled machine. What do you want? What's realistic? What can you agree upon? Can you keep up the newfound consistency of two great Sessions every week?

Mix it up in whatever way feels right: there might be some weeks when you have one Solo Session and a super creative and wild Long Love Engagement. On another week, you might be all about a Quickie and a BJ. You might even take an extended kid-free vacation, and challenge each other to cycle through all eight of the Sessions! Of course, there could also be other weeks when you may net out at a *big fat zero*. It's all good.

Try sitting down every Sunday night together, and sketching out your Sexy Session goals for the week. Keep communicating, and remember to practice the principles of priority, planning, flexibility, and follow-through. Also, keep trying new things in the Fantasy Fun Session, new locations for Playtime, a new scenario in which you Receive Pleasure. Continue to dig deeper with your partner, seeking sexier experiences to try. Pushing your limits will keep the spark alive and inspire your enthusiasm to stay on target. Always, *always* keep your eyes on the prize: a reignited chemistry and newly inspired sense of sexual intimacy and satisfaction. Now that you both have the tools to kick-start yourselves out of a sexual slump, keep using them. Above all else, keep reminding one another that couples who have consistent, communicative sex are just HAPPIER!

4. KEEP SEEKING OUT VISUAL STIMULATION

Whether you find yourself fantasizing over the phallic carrots at the grocery store, or you surf the web for a little dose of Eye Candy while you wait for your kid to finish their tutoring lesson, seek out sensual stimulation during your daily grind. In doing so, you'll keep your Mojo revving and fuel your sexual appetite.

When you see something that gives you a tingle down below, text your friends about it! Invite them to do the same. Seeing (and sharing) the "sexy" in your everyday mom life has the power to instantly arouse your senses and remind you of your sensual vitality as a woman. All you have to do is keep your eyes open to the turn-ons that already exist, and allow yourself to become excited and aroused as your imagination lights up. Then, when those thoughts start to turn you on, act on it. Grab your partner for a bonus Quickie, or sneak away for a Solo Session before you feed the kids their dinner.

5. BECOME AN ADVOCATE FOR MOMMY MOJO

One of the best ways to maintain your Mojo is to share the love and information with others. Just imagine if more and more moms maximized their Mojo and realized that they, too, are in control of their freedom, desires, libido, and satisfaction.

With this makeover experience under your belt, you have what it takes to spread the message of sexy self-confidence and a more satisfying relationship to the mamas all around you. Invite new moms into your Wild Women outings. Share which Sexy Sessions you and your spouse are taking on this week. Trade babysitting services so all your friends get to experience an Amazing Date Night out with their partners. Remember: With knowledge comes power and sharing that power with other moms in need will help keep the sexy revolution going.

6. SCORE QUICK HITS OF MOJO

Let's say you have the best of intentions for maintaining your Mojo, but life keeps getting in the way and you *never* practice any of the tools in this book ever again. It could happen! So how about choosing one quick hit of Mojo from this list and doing it whenever you can to feel sexier and more inspired:

- ♥ Dance in the mirror to your favorite music; get into your groove
- ♥ Go commando (even if it's just around the house!)
- ♥ Declutter your bedroom, light candles, and put out chocolates to nibble on
- ♥ Grab your partner for a passionate, unexpected kiss
- ♥ Do a handstand in lingerie
- ♥ Drop everything and do *exactly what you wanna do* for an hour
- ♥ Clean out your purse of all kid stuff: wrappers, juice boxes, snotty Kleenexes
- ♥ Talk about sex over coffee with your Mom Tribe
- ♥ Take a quick Mommy Pop-Out, no matter how short it is!
- ♥ Dress up in something sexy, even if there's no place to go
- ♥ Hide from your kids for ten minutes and meditate
- ♥ Go on a Moms' Night Out and flirt shamelessly
- ♥ Treat yourself to a new sex toy
- ♥ Take five minutes to primp in the mirror and tell yourself how sexy you are

- ♥ Dive into bed and give yourself a mind-blowing orgasm
- ♥ Write and post a Mojo Mantra on the refrigerator door
- ♥ Ask your partner for a sensual massage
- ♥ Leave the laundry to sit another day as an act of rebellion
- ♥ Mist yourself with your favorite scent
- ♥ Read an article about sex!
- ♥ Throw your schedule out the window and do something wildly fun instead
- ♥ Say YES to sex at midnight
- ♥ Say NO to overcommitting yourself
- ♥ Delegate as much housework as possible, as often as you can
- ♥ Tell yourself out loud what an amazing, sexy, powerful, youthful, and alive WOMAN YOU ARE!

Whatever you do, don't slip back into a distant last place on your priority list. And don't get comfortable where you are right now, either! Motherhood should be celebrated. Sexuality should be celebrated. And awakened sexuality in motherhood should be celebrated, too! So, keep kicking your Mojo up a notch . . . and then another notch and another. You got this, Mama!

My Wish For You

Dear Mama,

Something really amazing has happened here. You've committed to sensual self-discovery and invited authentic sexiness back into your relationship. You harnessed the power of your pussy and embraced pleasure as a means to create a luscious and satisfying experience of motherhood.

You've discovered that passion exists within your daily grind, that there is sizzling stimulation in your everyday routine just waiting for you to see it—and seize it. There is a wild, sensual woman that lives inside of you, and she wants you to continue to invite her out to play.

Investing in yourself this way means that you love yourself enough to nurture the sensual woman that you are, that you always have been. Because your little ones deserve a mama who knows how to take care of herself, too! You deserve all the freedom, fun, confidence, and bliss that you've brought into your world as both a mother and partner. I'm beyond proud of you!

My wish for you is to never forget just how beautiful, powerful, sensual, and interesting you are. To know that it is within your reach to fill yourself up every single day—to be bubbling over with love, passion, self-care, communication, and, of course, amazing orgasms. I want you to always remember that it is within your reach to keep your relationship brimming with desire, excitement, and deep intimate connection. Yes, Mama, you CAN be an incredible mom and wife and still have a sexy, turned-on life.

So keep practicing the tools in this book! They will remind you of that all of this is possible—even as the years go by.

And so today, and every day from now on, I invite you to celebrate yourself as a SEXY WOMAN . . . who just so also happens to be a mother. I invite you to know just how strong, loving, deserving, sexy, juicy, and truly amazing you are.

I invite you to honor yourself as:

- ♥ A kick-ass mother . . .
- ♥ A confident lover . . .
- ♥ An equal partner . . .
- ♥ An inspiring girlfriend . . .
- ♥ A smart, capable woman!

I want you to make every day as arousing, magical, creative, and pleasurable as possible—no matter how many dishes or diapers get in your way. Keep placing yourself higher and higher on your priority list, talk about sex with the other moms in your life, and make motherhood fun again!

Above all else, I urge you to give your best to your children and to your partner, while always making time to connect with yourself first as a woman. And with everything that you've learned in this book and how much you've evolved, I believe that your charged-up confidence and lit-up libido will lead you there—naturally.

All my love . . .
XOXO,
Dana

Acknowledgments

I want to begin by thanking YOU, my dear reader, for your willingness to evolve into the sexy mama you were born to be. I'm inspired by your rekindled desire—your courage, breakthroughs, and triumphs. I am honored to be on this journey with you, and I am here for you every step of the way.

I would also like to thank my mom, Barbara, who set an example for me of what sensual confidence and feminine vitality looks like in motherhood. And, of course, to my dad, who ingrained true grit and tenacity into the very core of my being.

To Andrea, my brilliant copy editor, thank you for your remarkable talent and endless patience with run-on sentences and overuse of italics. You were the glowing, golden angel on my shoulder throughout this whole process.

To Eileen, my agent and my friend. You've been my rock! Your support means the world to me.

To Anna, the super-nanny who helped care for the kids as I wrote this book. To trust someone with our children as much I trusted you is such a blessing. Words can't express my gratitude! And to Alejandra, who supported me as I finished and released this into the world. Thank you, thank you, thank you!

To my island Mom Tribe: Jamie, Rena, and Shannon. I couldn't have completed this book, or my time in St. Lucia, without your daily encouragement and love. I miss you!

To the rest of my Mom Tribe scattered across the world: Cameron, Katherine, Lauren, Dominika, Karine, Mimi, Jenny, Jess, and Meg. I love you. Motherhood is so much more inspiring with you in my life.

To all the moms I've worked with who've shared their true stories with me over the years—your names may have been changed, but you know who you are! Thank you for your honesty and enthusiasm to contribute your personal experiences with the women reading this book. You tested out my ideas and your courage, feedback, and continued friendship have made this book possible.

To the Viva Editions team, thank you for believing in the Mommy Mojo Makeover, and for your support, thoughtful edits, and encouragement.

To my kids, Rocky and Indie, I am who I am because of YOU. I work harder to fulfill my dreams so that you know you can achieve yours. Because of you, I wrote this book and found my calling. Because of you, our marriage is stronger. Becoming your mother is the best thing I have ever done, and will ever do, in my whole life.

And to Charlie, my epic husband, my greatest lover, my tenacious business partner, my very best friend, you are my most treasured gift in this life. Your support is the backbone of my success and our amazing, adventurous life together brings me happiness and experiences beyond my wildest dreams! Parenthood is one crazy ride, hard and amazing in ways we never could have expected, and I love that YOU are the one I get to experience it with. I'm forever crazy about you, forever grateful to you, and forever first in line to eat your delicious cooking—because it will always be way better than mine. XOXO, baby.

More Resources for Your Mommy Mojo

I believe that every mother wants, needs, and deserves to feel sexy, confident, and desirable. My hope is that you will use this book as an empowering tool to rediscover your own unique sexiness, to light up your mojo, and inspire you to create more satisfying experiences within motherhood, womanhood, and your relationship. Motherhood ain't easy . . . but together, I know we can make it *far more pleasurable!* I'm so grateful that my book has found its way into your world, and I'd love to continue our connection online.

Join my online community.
I have an ever-growing library of resources that you can access right now at www.DanaBMyers.com. Blogs, videos, actionable worksheets, and more are waiting for you! There you'll find all the ways to connect with me on social media and discover links to my additional teachings, workshops, and digital courses.

Get *Mojo motivation* delivered to your inbox.
Activating your Mommy Mojo in small, consistent ways can add up to major shifts in your sensuality and sexual satisfaction, and that's what my weekly newsletters are designed to help you do. Sign up

www.DanaBMyers.com to receive my free newsletters that'll inspire you to continue your makeover journey!

About the Author

DANA B. MYERS is an award-winning product developer, entrepreneur, author, and media personality. As Founder of Booty Parlor, Dana B. Myers has changed the lives of thousands of women by inspiring them to boost their sensual self-confidence and create sexier, more satisfying relationships.

Known for her frank yet empowering style, Dana helps her clients reclaim the power of their sensuality and sexual satisfaction through her coaching practice and live workshops. Her advice, and Booty Parlor's products, have been featured by *Marie Claire, Women's Health, Parents, Redbook, Nylon, Allure,* and the *Wall Street Journal.* Dana has appeared on *ABC Nightline, Good Morning America, Access Hollywood Live, The Wendy Williams Show,* and more.

Born and raised in Chicago, Dana earned a Master's Degree in Business & Entertainment from NYU. Having lived in Los Angeles, Brooklyn, and St. Lucia, she now resides in Miami with her husband and business partner, Charlie, and their two children, Rocky and Indie.

Become part of the #MommyMojo community at www.DanaBMyers.com.

 /DanaBMyers

 /danamyersxoxo

 /danamyersxoxo